George Alexopoulos

Siegfried Kasper

Hans-Jürgen Möller

Carmen Moreno

Guide to Assessment Scales in Major Depressive Disorder

George Alexopoulos
Cornell University, New York, USA

Siegfried Kasper
Medical University of Vienna, Austria

Hans-Jürgen Möller
Ludwig Maximilian University, Munich, Germany

Carmen Moreno
Complutense University, Madrid, Spain

Guide to Assessment Scales in Major Depressive Disorder

Contributors

Marta Bravo, Maria Mayoral, Alejandra Teresa Laorden

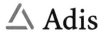

ISBN 978-3-319-04626-6/ISBN (eBook) 978-3-319-04627-3
DOI 10.1007/978-3-319-04627-3
Springer Cham Heidelberg New York Dordrecht London

Printed on acid-free paper

Springer is part of Springer Science+Business Media (www.springer.com)

Project editor: Katrina Dorn
Designer: Roland Codd

Contents

Author biographies

George Alexopoulos, MD, is SP Tobin and AM Cooper Professor of Psychiatry, founder and director of the Weill-Cornell Institute of Geriatric Psychiatry, and director of the Advanced Center for Interventions and Services Research in Geriatric Mood Disorders at Cornell University, New York, USA. Dr Alexopoulos received his MD from the National University of Athens, Greece, trained at New Jersey Medical School, and completed his psychiatric residency at Cornell University Medical College, where he completed a research fellowship in Psychobiology. Dr Alexopoulos has made fundamental contributions to the study of the biology of late-life depression including identifying brain mechanisms contributing to poor response to antidepressant drugs, development of new treatments for patients with depression and severe medical illnesses, and improving the practice model for the identification and treatment of depression in primary care. Dr Alexopoulos has served on the Board of Scientific Counselors of the National Institute of Mental Health and has received four consecutive Center Grant Awards from the National Institute of Mental Health and numerous individual grants. He has been the Director of the T32 NIMH Research Fellowship in Geriatric Mood Disorders since 1989. Dr Alexopoulos is a fellow of the American College of Neuropsychopharmacology, American College of Psychiatrists (ACP), and a Distinguished Life Fellow of the American Psychiatric Association (APA). He has received several awards, including an APA Presidential Commendation, the Research Award of the International College of American College of Geriatric Psychoneuropharmacology, the APA Greenberg Award, the ACP Geriatric Research Award, the Joseph Zubin Research Award of the American Psychopathological Association, the APA Distinguished Psychiatrist Lecturer Award, and the Senior Investigator's Award of the American Association for Geriatric Psychiatry. Dr Alexopoulos is the editor of the *International Journal of Geriatric Psychiatry* (Western Hemisphere) and has published more than 400 articles and book chapters.

Siegfried Kasper, MD is Professor of Psychiatry and Chairman of the Department of Psychiatry and Psychotherapy at the Medical University of Vienna, Austria. Dr Kasper serves/served on the executive committees and advisory boards of several national and international societies, such as the European College of Neuropsychopharmacology (ECNP) and the European Psychiatric Association (EPA). He has been elected to the Executive Committee of the International College of Neuropsychopharmacology (CINP) for the period of 2012 to 2016. He is Chair of the World Psychiatric Association (WPA) Section of Pharmacopsychiatry, President of the Austrian Society of Drug Safety in Psychiatry (ÖAMSP), and Past-President of the Austrian Society of Neuropsychopharmacology and Biological Psychiatry (ÖGPB). Dr Kasper is an Honorary Member of the Czech and Romanian Societies of Neuropsychopharmacology, the Hungarian Psychiatric Association, and a Fellow of the Royal College of Psychiatrists (UK) and Ukrainian Association of Psychiatry. Dr Kasper has been President of the 10th ECNP Congress , Chairman of the Local Organizing Committee of the WPA Thematic Conference, and Co-

Chair of the Local Organizing Committee of the WFSBP Congress. In 2009, he was President of the WFSBP Congress in Paris. In 2005, he was appointed Honorary Professor at the University of Hong Kong, China. From 2005 to 2009, Dr Kasper was President of the World Federation of Societies of Biological Psychiatry (WFSBP) and was appointed as Honorary President of the WFSBP in 2013. Dr Kasper serves on editorial boards of numerous learned journals, including *Lancet Psychiatry, Journal of Clinical Psychiatry, CNS Spectrums, Journal of Affective Disorders, Pharmacopsychiatry, European Archives of Psychiatry,* and *Neuroscience.* He is Editor-in-Chief of the *World Journal of Biological Psychiatry* and the *International Journal of Psychiatry in Clinical Practice,* and Field Editor of the *International Journal of Neuropsychopharmacology.* Dr Kasper has published over 1000 ISI-listed publications and more than 200 book chapters.

Hans-Jürgen Möller, MD, is Emeritus Professor at the Department of Psychiatry, Ludwig Maximilian University, Munich, Germany, where he was Chairman and Professor of Psychiatry from 1994 to 2012. He has worked in the field of psychiatry for more than 40 years. After obtaining his Doctor of Medical Science in 1972, he completed postgraduate training in psychiatry at the Max Planck Institute of Psychiatry in Munich. From 1980 to 1988 he was Professor of Psychiatry at Munich Technical University and from 1988 to 1994 full Professor of Psychiatry and Chairman of the Department of Psychiatry at the University of Bonn. His main scientific contributions include clinical and neurobiological research into psychiatry, schizophrenia and depression and clinical psychopharmacology. He has written and co-authored over 1,100 publications, including numerous original articles (Hirsch Factor 68) and several books. He is co-editor of *European Archives of Psychiatry and Clinical Neuroscience* and *Psychopharmakotherapie,* founding editor and former chief editor of *The World Journal of Biological Psychiatry* and holds positions on the editorial boards of several national and international psychiatric journals. He has been a member of the executive committees of many national and international psychiatric societies. He was President of the World Federation of Societies of Biological Psychiatry (WFSBP), President of the European Psychiatric Association (EPA) and Chairman of the World Psychiatric Association (WPA) Section on Pharmacopsychiatry. Currently, he is Past-President of the Collegium Internationale Neuro-Psychopharmacologicum (CINP). He has received numerous awards including the WPA Jean Delay Prize and the WFSBP Lifetime Achievement Award.

Carmen Moreno, MD, PhD, is a Child Psychiatrist and Associate Professor of the Gregorio Marañón Psychiatry Department, Complutense University School of Medicine, Madrid, Spain. Dr. Moreno completed her MD and PhD degrees at Autónoma University and Complutense University in Madrid, and a Research Fellowship in Child and Adolescent Psychiatry at Columbia University, New York, USA. Dr. Moreno has focused her career on early-onset psychiatric disorders, mainly affective and psychotic disorders, and recently, also other neurodevelopmental disorders. She is recognized by her studies in raising awareness of the misdiagnosis of bipolar disorder in children and adolescents. She has authored more than 30 peer-reviewed publications. Her efforts are now focused on understanding the role of inflammation and oxidative stress on early-onset psychiatric disorders, and towards development of new treatment interventions.

1. Introduction to assessment in depression

Siegfried Kasper, Hans-Jürgen Möller

Introduction

The diagnosis of depression has been revised over the past decade in accordance with the International Statistical Classification (ICD-10) and Diagnostic and Statistical Manual of Mental Disorders (DSM)-5 diagnostic criteria [1,2]. While these publications give a framework for the classification of mental disorders, there is also a necessity for a multidimensional approach, which can be obtained by using assessment scales for syndromes across different psychiatric categories. It is worth noting that these scales cannot be used for establishing diagnosis but are helpful for grading the severity of the condition irrespective of the diagnostic category, as well as enabling treatment plans for psychopharmacological and psychotherapeutic methods.

Different psychometric rating scales have been used for evaluating psychotropic agents within and across diagnostic categories. Although this indicates the validity of the scales used, it does not mean that they are necessarily the most sensitive scales for certain indications. One example is the Hamilton Depression Rating Scale for Depression (HAM-D), which can overemphasize sedative antidepressants because there are three items for sleep disturbances (in contrast to the Montgomery-Åsberg Rating Scale for Depression [MADRS] with only one item relating to sleep parameters) [3,4]. It should be emphasized that many rating scales do not adequately reflect our current understanding of the phenomenology of the disorders (eg, male depression with higher levels of aggression), which may change as continued research leads to the discovery of new neurobiological entities.

Multivariate analysis

Multivariate statistical analysis (factor and cluster analysis) of the data obtained from rating scales may be used to derive factors. These factors identify groups of individual symptoms that tend to occur together. If we consider that the term 'clinical syndrome' generally refers to a group of symptoms that frequently occur in combination, it becomes apparent that the

© Springer International Publishing Switzerland 2014
G. Alexopoulos et al., *Guide to Assessment Scales in Major Depressive Disorder*,
DOI 10.1007/978-3-319-04627-3_1

factors extracted from rating scales relating to mental state are conceptually identical to clinical syndromes. Multivariate analysis of the data obtained by using different multidimensional psychiatric rating scales in different samples of patients has tended to repeatedly generate the same factors or symptom clusters [5–10]:

- paranoid hallucinatory syndrome;
- manic syndrome;
- depressive syndrome;
- apathetic syndrome;
- hypochondriac syndrome;
- phobic-obsessive syndrome; and
- amnesiac syndrome.

The factor structure of some well-developed observer rated scales has also been shown to remain relatively stable across different studies and, for many of the factors, even across repeated measurements over the course of treatment [11–13]. This invariability in the structure of factors across different samples and time points is an important aspect of the validity of a scale (factorial validity).

Limitations of rating scales

It is important to bear in mind that the items included in factors or dimensions may vary greatly between scales, even if the names of the factors or dimensions are the same. Also, the correlation might differ quite considerably between the scores of analogous factors or dimensions of a scale and the total scores of two scales focusing on the same clinical phenomenon (eg, depression). Possible consequences include discrepancies such as efficacy results in antidepressants trials; for example, in a study on lamotrigine in bipolar depression, only the MADRS ratings showed a statistically significant difference between lamotrigine and placebo, while the HAM-D ratings, which were defined as the primary outcome measure, did not [14]. Therefore, careful thought must be put into the selection of a scale for a clinical study.

The development of standardized rating scales, both observer and self-rating, is a time-consuming, long-lasting process that includes several complex procedures to determine validity and reliability, among other aspects [15]. This is one of the main reasons that only a few psychometrically well-validated scales are widely available. However, the increasingly popular trend to generate and publish new rating scales, eg, in the context of certain research projects and often after a short development period, is not a recommended approach to for advancing the field. For example, a scale cannot be designed by simply taking the DSM-5 or ICD-10 symptoms of depression, providing a scoring rubric, investigating a sample of depressed patients, and then calculating the correlations between the total scores of the new and the established scales. When assessing correlations with another scale, for example, it is very important that the scale is evaluated in a sample of patients at all levels of severity (mild, moderate, and severe). This is especially important if the new scale is a self-rating scale that is to be validated through its correlation with an observer rating scale, because the correlation depends on severity. Such comparisons of self-rating and observer rating scales should also include correlations over time because cross-sectional correlations can vary at different points in time.

Nevertheless, such unprofessionally developed instruments sometimes attract attention for a while, until the deficiencies, such as lack of validity or reliability, become clear. Interestingly, psychometrically well-developed standardized rating instruments, including the WHO instruments for the assessment of depressive disorders [16], sometimes do not gain acceptance even when they have been carefully tested internationally; the reasons for this phenomenon are unclear.

Thus, the development of new rating scales for psychopharmacological research is often hampered because measures of efficacy using established scales are required by international regulatory agencies to approve a new medication; outcome data from a new rating instrument are regarded as supplemental evidence. Another problematic point is the possible overlap between treatment-emergent side effects of psychoactive drugs with symptoms of psychiatric disorders, which can only be disentangled by sound knowledge of both the disease as well as the pharmacodynamic and pharmacokinetic properties of the compounds under evaluation.

Using assessment scales in clinical practice

Despite these limitations, it is evident that the available scales for depression, which are now part of a standardized approach for assessment of most major mental disorder conditions, are helpful for communication between patients and clinicians and aid in the evaluation of treatment efficacy, from both an individual and statistical approach. Available scales can be categorized as observer- or self-rating scales and it is evident that both approaches are needed in order to obtain detailed information about the patient and the treatment process. In Chapter 2, these approaches are described along with the most commonly used scales for depression. For example, the HAM-D and the MADRS are evaluated in detail and their clinical and scientific cross-sectional and longitudinal utility are discussed. It is emphasized that self-rating scales may have a higher variance than observer-rated scales, which often necessitates larger trial sample sizes of the observed population in order to achieve statistically significant effects.

A series of fully structured interview schedules and diagnostic instruments developed in the last decade allow ICD-10 and DSM-5 diagnoses to be generated: the Composite Diagnostic Interview [17,18], the Structured Clinical Interview for DSM [19,20], and the PSE-based Schedules for Clinical Assessment in Neuropsychiatry [21,22]. Overall, these instruments seem likely to lead to a considerable increase in inter-rater reliability in the assessment of mental states and in diagnostic classification. However, as mentioned above, these fully structured instruments are often too time-consuming and expensive for everyday clinical use. They are primarily indicated for diagnosing depression or different types of depression, and not simply for assessing the severity of depression or the course of severity.

Use of scales in pediatric depression

The assessment of pediatric depression is a challenge, as the apparent symptoms are often a topic for interpretation rather than assessment. Chapter 4 describes the different scales used for pediatric depression and discusses their usefulness for establishing treatment options for this group of patients. Early and accurate diagnosis is especially important to this population because longer duration of untreated illness in children and adolescents has been linked to more frequent recurrences which, together with emerging difficulties in the development of psychosocial and emotional skills, can lead to poor outcomes [23].

Use of scales in elderly depression

The assessment of depression in geriatric patients is described in Chapter 5. Various factors complicate the assessment of depression in cognitively impaired patients or those with dementia because symptoms of depression can overlap with behavioral manifestations such as apathy and loss of initiative. Furthermore, in patients with dementia, depressive symptoms may fluctuate over time or fail to meet the criteria for intensity, duration, or functional impact required for a diagnosis of major depression (eg, DSM-5) [1]. Therefore, when assessing symptoms in late-life depression, more specific scales such as the Dementia Mood Assessment Scale or the Cornell Scale for Depression in Dementia may be considered [24,25].

The scales reviewed in this book reflect the most important contemporary assessment tools used in depression, including those scales for populations spanning the lifespan. The aim of this book is to provide a clinically relevant resource that a busy clinician can pragmatically use to evaluate the patient. Additionally, the information in the book will enhance understanding of the psychosocial situation and aid in interpreting the responses a patient and/or their relatives give to describe the patient's current mental state.

References

1   World Health Organization (WHO). International Classification of Diseases. WHO website. www.who.int/classifications/icd/en/. Accessed August 29, 2014.
2   American Psychiatric Association (APA). *Diagnostic and Statistical Manual of Mental Disorders.* 5th edn. Arlington, VA: American Psychiatric Publishing; 2013.
3   Hamilton M. A rating scale for depression. *J Neurol Neurosurg Psychiatry.* 1960;23:56-62.
4   Montgomery SA, Åsberg M. A new depression scale designed to be sensitive to change. *Br J Psychiatry.* 1979;134:382-389.
5   Cairns V, Faltermaier T, Wittchen HU, et al. Some problems concerning the reliability and structure of the scales in the inpatient multidimensional psychiatric scale (IMPS). *Arch Psychiatr Nervenkr.* 1982; 232:395-406.
6   Cairns V, von Zerssen D, Stutte KH et al. The stability of the symptom groupings in the Inpatient Multidimensional Psychiatric Scale (IMPS). *J Psychiatr Res.* 1982;17:19-28.
7   Gebhardt R, Pietzcker A, Freudenthal K, et al. [Building syndromes in the AMP-system (author's transl)]. *Arch Psychiatr Nervenkr.* 1981;231:93-109.
8   Lorr M, Mc ND, Klett CJ, et al. Evidence of ten psychotic syndromes. *J Consult Psychol.* 1962; 26:185-189.

9 Mombour W. [Frequency of symptoms in psychiatric illnesses. A comparative investigation with two rating scales (IMPS and AMP-scale)--psychological-pathological findings (author's transl)]. *Arch Psychiatr Nervenkr.* 1974;219:133-152.

10 Mombour W. [Syndromes in psychiatric illnesses. A comparative investigation with two rating scales (IMPS and AMP-scale) (author's transl)]. *Arch Psychiatr Nervenkr.* 1974;219:331-350.

11 Baumann U, Stieglitz RD. Testmanual zum AMDPSystem. Empirische Studien zur Psychopathologie. Berlin: Springer; 1983.

12 Moller HJ, Hacker H. Study concerning the sample dependency and temporal variance of the factor structure in the Inpatient Multidimensional Psychiatric Scale. *Psychopathology.* 1988;21:281-290.

13 Steinmeyer EM, Moller HJ. Facet theoretic analysis of the Hamilton-D scale. *J Affect Disord.* 1992;25:53-61.

14 Calabrese JR, Bowden CL, Sachs GS et al. A double-blind placebo-controlled study of lamotrigine monotherapy in outpatients with bipolar I depression. Lamictal 602 Study Group. *J Clin Psychiatry.* 1999;60:79-88.

15 Moller HJ. Standardised rating scales in psychiatry: methodological basis, their possibilities and limitations and descriptions of important rating scales. *World J Biol Psychiatry.* 2009;10:6-26.

16 Jablensky N, Sartorius N, Gulbinat W et al. The WHO instruments for the assessment of depressive disorders. In: *Assessment of Depression.* Edited by Sartorius N, Ban TA. Berlin: Springer; 1986;61-81.

17 Wittchen HU, Semmler G. Composite International Diagnostic Interview (CIDI, version 1.0). Weinheim: Beltz; 1991.

18 Wittchen HU, Semmler G. Composite International Diagnostic Interview (CIDI, version 2.0). Weinheim: Beltz; 1997.

19 Wittchen HU, Wunderlich U, Gruschwitz S et al. *Strukturiertes Klinisches Interview für DSM-IV (SKID).* Göttingen: Hogrefe; 1997.

20 Wittchen HU, Zaudig M, Spengler P. Wie zuverlässig ist operationalisierte Diagnostik? Die Test-Retest Reliabilität des Strukturierten Interviews für DSM-III-R. *Z Klin Psychol.* 1991;20:136-153.

21 World Health Organization (WHO). Schedule for the clinical assessment in neuropsychiatry. Geneva: WHO; 1991.

22 WHO. Schedule for the clinical assessment in neuropsychiatry. Version 2.1. Geneva: WHO; 1999.

23 Cullen K, Klimes-Dougan B, Kumra S, Schulz SC. Paediatric major depressive disorder: neurobiology and implications for early intervention. *Early Interv Psychiatry.* 2009;3:178-188.

24 Sunderland T, Hill JL, Lawlor BA, Molchan SE. NIMH Dementia Mood Assessment Scale (DMAS). *Psychopharmacol Bull.* 1988;24:747-753.

25 Alexopoulos GS, Abrams RC, Young RC, Shamoian CA. Cornell Scale for Depression in Dementia. *Biol Psychiatry.* 1988;23:271-284.

2. Observer rating scales

Hans-Jürgen Möller

Introduction

Observer rating scales (also called observer rating scales, observer scales, or clinical scales) relate to past or current behavior and experiences [1]. These standardized scales are used to rate the extent of psychopathological phenomena and may focus on a single aspect of psychopathology (unidimensional scales) or on several aspects (multidimensional scales). For example, to evaluate only the severity of depression, a unidimensional scale is sufficient. To assess other symptom dimensions, such as anxiety and obsessive-compulsive and psychotic symptoms, a multidimensional scale or a combination of different unidimensional scales is indicated. In a long-term study on patients with depression, a broad range multidimensional scale like the Association for Methodology and Documentation in Psychiatry (AMDP) system [2] might be indicated in order to record mood switches (eg, to manic or psychotic symptoms), despite the focus of the study being on depression [3]. It should be noted that even if the name of a scale appears to indicate that it is unidimensional and focuses on one syndrome or disorder, the scale is very often not actually unidimensional, but multidimensional; this is true for the Hamilton Depression Rating Scale (HAM-D) [4,5].

General aspects of observer rating scales

For each aspect of psychopathology, the assessment may be based on a global rating or on different elements within the aspect being assessed (eg, individual symptoms of the depressive syndrome). In the latter case, the overall score of the instrument is obtained by summing values for these different elements.

Standardization

Assessment or rating scales do not have a uniform level of standardization. Standardization for most of these instruments is limited to providing guidelines that describe the items and the

© Springer International Publishing Switzerland 2014
G. Alexopoulos et al., *Guide to Assessment Scales in Major Depressive Disorder*,
DOI 10.1007/978-3-319-04627-3_2

categories used to assess them and specifying a method to analyze the assessments. Generally, a total score or summary scores (consisting of a total score and subscores) are calculated. For some scales, a time frame and the framework in which the observation should take place are stipulated for the assessment. In the latter case, the instrument is referred to as a fully structured or standardized interview. The more extensive the standardization procedures, the more reliable an assessment instrument generally becomes. However, a highly standardized instrument tends to become less practicable. As a result, for pragmatic reasons the non-fully structured instruments (ie, the typical clinical rating scales such as the HAM-D) are preferred to fully structured instruments in both everyday clinical use and research because they can be completed after a routine psychiatric interview. The inter-rater reliability of these simpler clinical rating scales is lower than that of fully structured assessment instruments. However, this disadvantage can be at least partially compensated for by systematic joint training of raters, as is the case in clinical trials for drug evaluation.

Symptom assessment

In observer rating instruments, psychopathological phenomena (symptoms) are identified by trained raters (eg, doctors, psychologists, care staff, lay people trained to administer the instrument) or by relevant others (eg, partner, relatives, friends). The assessment refers to the behavior and/or experience of the patient and is based on the rater's own observations, information given by the patient or both. Observer rating scales need to be constructed in a way that makes them suitable for the interviewers who will administer them. Thus, some scales are designed for doctors or psychologists trained in psychiatry (eg, Montgomery-Åsberg Depression Rating Scale [MADRS] [6]), while others are designed for care staff trained in psychiatry or for patients' relatives.

Observer rating scales mainly focus on the psychopathological state. The aim of the scale may be to classify each individual wholly as a 'case' or 'non-case' [7], record specific aspects of the patient's mental state [8,9], or assess the whole spectrum of psychopathology (eg, AMDP system). The more syndromes that are represented in a scale, the wider the range of its potential applications will be. For example, a comprehensive multidimensional scale like the AMDP system [2] covers a wide range of symptoms and syndromes characteristic for different mental disorders, including depression. Such a comprehensive scale is useful as part of a clinical basic documentation system that covers all kinds of patients, for example, or in a long-term follow-up study in which patients can be expected to switch into different syndromes (eg, from mania into bipolar depression and vice versa; or from non-psychotic to psychotic major depression and vice versa). However, in order to address specific issues for which even a comprehensive scale does not collect enough data (eg, detailed aspects of suicidal behavior), a comprehensive rating scale should be combined with other specific observer rating scales (eg, the Columbia-Suicide Severity Rating Scale) [10].

When professionally trained assessors administer observer rating instruments, they decide how much weight to put on the information the patient gives. In addition, observable changes are taken into account in the rating, for example an improvement in general behavior and demeanor, even if the patient gives no clear report of this improvement. An advantage of this expert assessment is that it reduces the scope for inaccurate assessments resulting from distortions in patients' perception of themselves. However, it does introduce the risk of distortion related to the assessor (rater bias). Systematic distortion in the assessor's observations [11] can result from the following factors in particular:

- **Rosenthal effect:** The assessor's expectations influence the result of the assessment; tendency on the part of the assessor to systematically over- or under-rate the degree of disturbance;
- **Halo effect:** The results of the assessment of one characteristic are influenced by the assessor's knowledge of the patient's other characteristics or by the overall impression made by the patient; and/or
- **Logical errors:** The result of the assessment is influenced by assessors reporting only those detailed observations that make sense to them in the context of their theoretical and logical preconceptions. These errors may be partially compensated for by combining observer rating scales with self-rated scales [1].

Most rating scales allow the current mental state to be described. When performed at intervals, they can also be used to examine changes over time, although they were not originally specifically developed for such use. During further development of the scales, changes over time were rather studied with sophisticated statistical analyses focusing on the item development and internal structure of the item association over time and whether the total score of all items or a subset of items always reflect severity in the same way [12,13].

Of interest, especially in the context of psychopharmacological studies, is the administration of observer rating scales like the HAM-D with a telephone-based interactive voice recording system (IVRS), rather than in a face-to-face interview [14–16]. The IVRS can increase reliability and is cost-effective. However, when administered via such a system, the HAM-D is technically no longer being used as a true observer rating scale (ie, although information given by the patient is being assessed, the expert interpretation of this information and clinical observation of depression-related behavior changes such as facial expression are lacking). When used with this new approach, the process becomes similar to a self-rating procedure, with all of its limitations (see Chapter 3).

Examples of observer rating scales for depression

Several observer rating scales for depression are available; the most traditional and probably the first to be developed, the HAM-D, has been in use for more than 50 years [4,17]. Nearly all antidepressants have been evaluated on the basis of the HAM-D. Although often criticized for several reasons [18], this scale has remained popular for both the evaluation of antidepressants in clinical studies and for other clinical purposes [19]. This scale has an obvious face validity for all doctors trained in psychiatry when they consider its rich coverage of clinically relevant depression symptoms. In comparison, the MADRS is a more modern scale that has certain advantages such as its shortness (10 items), sensitivity to change, and lack of bias for sedating antidepressants. This lack of bias has resulted in the MADRS being used in many drug trials evaluating modern antidepressants.

Several other depression scales are available [1] that are used under certain conditions or in certain countries, but none are used as widely as the HAM-D and MADRS. Some depression scales were developed in the USA that tended to be primarily based on the symptoms in the Diagnostic and Statistical Manual of Mental Disorders (DSM)-IV description of major depression, for example [20,21]. Although these scales have demonstrated their clinical usefulness in a few larger North American studies such as the Sequenced Treatment Alternatives to Relieve Depression or Systematic Treatment Enhancement Program for Bipolar Disorder, they have not yet become globally accepted. However, the Inventory of Depressive Symptomatology from Rush et al [20] and its respective short version, the Quick Inventory of Depressive Symptomatology [22], might gain wider acceptance in the future. The HAM-D and MADRS are described in detail below. The description includes information on how to use each scale and how it was constructed and psychometrically evaluated, which demonstrates the quality standards of the scale.

In addition to the mental state, domains such as social adjustment may also be measured by observer rating scales. The assessment of social functioning is a useful additional outcome dimension because it helps obtain a full picture of a patient's problems and burdens. Examples include:

- Social Adjustment Scale (SAS) [23];
- Social Interview Schedule (SIS) [24,25];
- World Health Organization Disability Assessment Schedule (WHODAS) [26];
- Global Assessment Scale (GAS) [27];
- Social and Occupational Functioning Assessment Scale (SOFAS) [28]; and
- Personal and Social Performance Scale [29]

The dimension of social functioning is complementary to the assessment of depressive symptoms; both ratings are only partially intercorrelated, depending on the respective dimension of psychopathology and social functioning [30].

Featured scale: Hamilton Rating Scale for Depression

The HAM-D [4,5,9] was one of the first observer rating scales for depression to gain worldwide acceptance, although its weaknesses have been increasingly criticized [31,32]. The item scoring sheets of the original 17-item version and the 24-item version of this scale are shown in Tables 2.1 and 2.2 (see Appendix A for the full scale) [33,34].

How to use the Hamilton Rating Scale for Depression

This observer rating scale is designed to be used by doctors or psychologists trained in psychiatry and with sufficient clinical experience. The rater evaluates the severity of the

Scoring sheet for the original, 17-item version of the Hamilton Depression (HAM-D) Rating Scale

Number	Symptom	Score
1*	Depressed mood	0–4
2*	Low self-esteem, guilt	0–4
3	Suicidal thoughts	0–4
4	Insomnia: initial	0–2
5	Insomnia: middle	0–2
6	Insomnia: late	0–2
7*	Work and interests	0–4
8*	Psychomotor retardation	0–4
9	Psychomotor agitation	0–4
10*	Anxiety, psychic	0–4
11	Anxiety, somatic	0–4
12	Gastrointestinal symptoms (appetite)	0–2
13*	Somatic symptoms, general	0–2
14	Sexual disturbances	0–2
15	Hypochondriasis (somatization)	0–4
16	Insight	0–3
17	Weight loss	0–2
	Total score:	0–53

Table 2.1 Scoring sheet for the original, 17-item version of the Hamilton Depression (HAM-D) Rating Scale. The time frame (window) is the past 3 days. *Depression factor. Adapted with permission from Hamilton [4,34] ©BMJ.

symptoms on the basis of information obtained during a clinical interview. Additional information obtained from relatives, friends, nurses and others may also be taken into consideration to enrich or correct the information given by the patient [34]. The interview, which is performed like a typical free or non-standardized psychiatric exploration, should last about 30 minutes to allow time to cover all the relevant points. The scale is intended to measure the severity of symptoms, not minor fluctuations, and therefore the patient's condition during the past few days or the past week should be considered.

To increase inter-rater reliability and to ensure that the scale is administered correctly (ie, that the items are correctly understood and rated), new users should receive brief training from raters experienced in using the scale. In research studies, either all patients should be assessed by two raters, who should discuss discrepant assessments after the rating, or the whole group of investigators should be given a formal rater training.

The scale measures individual depressive symptoms and their overall severity (reflected in the total score). Sequential HAM-D ratings are often used to assess the course of depression, for example in antidepressant studies. Experience has shown that ratings should generally not

Scoring sheet for the 24-item version of the Hamilton Depression (HAM-D) Rating Scale

Number	Symptom	Range	Score
1	Depressed mood	0–4	
2	Low self-esteem, guilt	0–4	
3	Suicidal thoughts	0–4	
4	Insomnia: initial	0–2	
5	Insomnia: middle	0–2	
6	Insomnia: late	0–2	
7	Work and interests	0–4	
8	Psychomotor retardation	0–4	
9	Psychomotor agitation	0–4	
10	Anxiety, psychic	0–4	
11	Anxiety, somatic	0–4	
12	Gastrointestinal symptoms (appetite)	0–2	
13	Somatic symptoms, general	0–2	
14	Sexual disturbances	0–2	
15	Hypochondriasis (somatization)	0–4	
16	Insight	0–2	
17	Weight loss	0–2	
18	Diurnal variation	0–2	
19	Depersonalization and derealization	0–4	
20	Paranoid symptoms	0–3	
21	Obsessional and compulsive symptoms	0–2	
22	Helplessness	0–4	
23	Hopelessness	0–4	
24	Worthlessness	0–4	
		Total score:	(0–75)

Table 2.2 Scoring sheet for the 24-item version of the Hamilton Depression (HAM-D) Rating Scale. Adapted with permission from Hamilton [4,33] ©BMJ.

be repeated at intervals shorter than 7 days. At repeat interviews, questions about changes in symptoms should be avoided. Also, before interviewing a patient, interviewers should not review the results of the previous rating.

The original scale contains 17 items [4], but 21- and 24-item scales were later developed [33]. Nevertheless, the original 17-item scale is used in and recommended for most psychopharmacological studies. Publications should always give details of the particular version of the scale that was used in a study because the score ranges for some items can vary. If no specific version is named, the reader can assume that the standard version was applied.

The degree of symptom severity is operationally defined for most of the items, which means that the rater must make the assessment on the basis of the content of specific statements and the tone, facial expression and gestures of the patient during the interview; the remaining items depend on a subjective selection of one of a number of levels of severity ranging from 'absent' to 'severe' or 'incapacitating'. Most of the items have a three-level score (0–2), the remaining ones a four- (0–3) or five-level (0–4) score, depending on the version of the scale being used. Symptom severity and frequency of symptoms should both be considered in the scoring. The total score of the HAM-D-17 ranges from 0–52 or 53 (depending on the version used), that of the HAM-D-21 from 0–64 and that of the HAM-D-24 from 0–76.

Quality and characteristics of the Hamilton Rating Scale for Depression

From a clinical standpoint, the type and spectrum of items characterizing depression seems prima facie meaningful: the items cover the traditional concept of depression, primarily the concept of endogenous depression, and are not influenced by the modern diagnostic classification systems. Somatic symptoms are more broadly represented than affective and cognitive symptoms. Some symptoms such as retardation (item 8) are relatively broad and include cognition, language, and motor activity. Symptoms typical for atypical depression such as hypersomnia and increased appetite or weight cannot be assessed because the scale only asks about changes in the opposite direction (ie, insomnia, reduced appetite, and weight loss). It is questionable whether the characteristic 'diurnal variations', which is included in the 21- and 24-item versions, should actually result in a higher depression score. The inclusion of this item can lead to contradictions in the diagnosis of the course of the disease because clinical experience shows that the most severe endogenous depressions often show no diurnal variations at first and that these only occur upon improvement of the severe depressive mood. The fact that three items rate sleep disorders (insomnia early, middle, and late) leads to an efficacy bias in antidepressant studies in favor of sedating or sleep-inducing antidepressants. Experts have discussed whether the slight efficacy advantage of tricyclic antidepressants over selective serotonin reuptake inhibitors (SSRIs) found in some studies and in meta-analyses might have been due to a bias of the HAM-D to capture sleep-inducing, sedating, and anxiolytic properties [35–37].

In addition to the possibility to calculate a total score, factor scores can also be calculated during the final analysis [4]. However, the results of factor analytical evaluations of the scale resulted in different solutions of 2 to 6 factors (which is not unusual for other rating scales in psychiatry) [4,9,38].

The inter-rater reliability is high to very high, at least for the total score, depending on the experience and training of the raters [4,39,40]. The retest reliability is also high [41].

Suggestions were made to define items and assessment criteria more explicitly, in order to increase the inter-rater reliability [42]. Consequently, a Structured Interview Guide was developed for the HAM-D (SIG-H) [41]; the guide has become quite well accepted in Anglo-American countries. However, when the interview guide is used, the HAM-D can no longer be seen as a rating scale but rather as a fully structured interview. As a result, it becomes more time consuming and no longer fits into the typical communication situation with the patient in a clinical setting and thus induces a somewhat artificial situation.

The HAM-D total score correlates well with the Clinical Global Impression rating of depression and with the total score of other depression scales, indicating its convergent validity [43–45]. As for discriminant validity, the HAM-D correlates moderately well with anxiety scales but the discrimination could be better. However, this finding is similar to that for other depression scales and has been a point of general criticism [46].

The sensitivity of the HAM-D to detect antidepressant-induced changes has been demonstrated in numerous antidepressant studies [47,48] (Figure 2.1) and, recently, in psychotherapy studies [49,50]. The good sensitivity to change can be interpreted as a strong indicator of validity. Reference values for various clinical samples are available [34], but norm values from a representative healthy population are not, as is also the case for most other clinical observer scales. A literature review of control groups in clinical studies of depression reported a mean HAM-D-17 score of 3.2 (SD 3.2) among healthy control individuals [51].

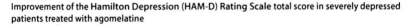

Improvement of the Hamilton Depression (HAM-D) Rating Scale total score in severely depressed patients treated with agomelatine

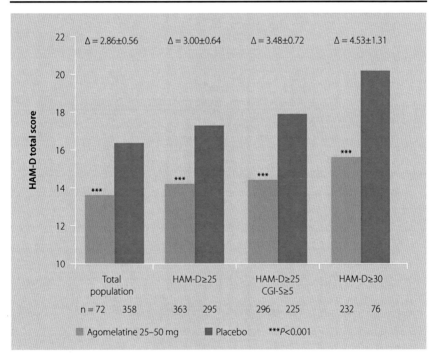

Figure 2.1 Improvement of the Hamilton Depression (HAM-D) Rating Scale total score in severely depressed patients treated with agomelatine. Dose of 25–50 mg/day for 6–8 weeks (meta-analysis of three positive studies) according to three severity criteria (HAM-D ≥25; HAM-D ≥25 and CGI-S ≥5; HAM-D ≥30). Reproduced with permission from Montgomery and Kasper [48] ©Lippincott, Williams and Wilkins.

Some additional problems of the scale still remain unresolved; for example, it does not record certain diagnostically specific areas that are partially included in other depression scales, such as the Inventory of Depressive Symptomatology (IDS) [28] (which includes symptoms of atypical depression) and, therefore, proves to be unsatisfactory for some subtypes of depression. The IDS is an extended version of the HAM-D and includes all DSM symptoms of major depression. It has 28 items (a more recent version has 30 items) and is available as an observer rating (IDS-C) and self-rated (IDS-SR) scale [52,53].

The HAM-D was subjected to critical test-theoretical analyses, including some performed according to the Rasch model and the facet analytical model, in order to investigate its homogeneity and the stability of the factor structure in repeated measurements during treatment and to find a minimal number of items that adequately reflect severity at different times [20,21,54]. The analyses resulted in a list of unidimensional core items. On the basis of this search for core items with optimal psychometric properties, short versions of the HAM-D were developed to assess depressive symptom severity:

- the Bech six-item version [55];
- a similar six-item version suggested by Maier and Philipp [56]; and
- a seven-item version of the HAM-D (HAM-D-7; [57,58]).

The Bech six-item version showed that this approach might lead to better results than the full-length version of the HAM-D in terms of differentiating antidepressant effects from those of placebo [59]. Other studies also found positive results for the Bech six-item version and other similar short versions [60,61]. Faries et al [62] and Entsuah et al [63] suggested that the use of such an unidimensional short scale requires fewer patients than the full HAM-D-17 scale. Also, such a scale may better detect the real antidepressant effect, independent of sedative and anxiolytic properties of the antidepressant [35]. On the basis of further analyses and clinical reflections, the Bech-Rafaelsen Melancholia Scale was developed (BRMES) [21,64], which consists of 11 items, 6 of which are in the Bech six-item version of the HAM-D.

For pragmatic and other reasons, self-rating versions of the original HAM-D were developed (eg, the Caroll Self-rating Scale for Depression [CDRS] and the Hamilton Depression Inventory [HDI] [65,66]). The latter scale has additional items and increased application possibilities, including a PC version [67] and an interactive voice response (IVR) version [68]. Self-rating versions were also developed from abbreviated versions [33,69].

In addition to reporting mean score changes, drug treatment studies in depression have increasingly focused on using remission as a relevant categorical efficacy criterion. In accordance with Frank et al [70], Rush et al [53] found on the basis of receiver operating characteristic (ROC) analyses of data from patients with major depression, healthy controls, and remitted patients that a HAM-D-17 score ≤7 (which corresponds to a HAM-D-7 score ≤3; [57]) is a meaningful criterion for remission [53]. The ACNP Task Force [71] recommended that if the HAM-D-17 scale is used, a score of ≤7 or ≤5 should be used as the criterion for remission. However, recent evidence supports the use of even more stringent remission criterion scores for both the HAM-D and MADRS scales [72]. A criticism of the use of response (in the common definition: 50% reduction from the baseline score) as an outcome measure is that it can identify a highly heterogeneous population of patients. However, defining remission with the suggested HAM-D-17 cut-off scores or even more stringent ones identifies populations of remitters that are as heterogeneous as the population of responders in terms of psychosocial impairment [73,74]. Patients with a HAM-D-17 score ≤2, for example, show better psychological functioning than those with scores of 3 to 7 [75,76].

Featured scale: Montgomery-Åsberg Depression Rating Scale

Although the HAM-D is still widely accepted and supported by a long tradition and enormous database in terms of psychometric evaluation and repeated use in all kinds of studies, the MADRS [6] is becoming an increasingly important observer rating scale thanks to its conciseness, better definition of items, ease of use, and modern approach to test construction (according to the principle of sensitivity to change). The sensitivity to change aspect seems to support its use in treatment-related studies. Contrary to the HAM-D, which covers a broad spectrum of depressive symptoms, the MADRS includes only the following ten items:

- apparent sadness;
- reported sadness;
- inner tension;
- reduced sleep;
- reduced appetite;
- concentration difficulties;
- lassitude;
- inability to feel;
- pessimistic thoughts; and
- suicidal thoughts.

How to use the Montgomery-Åsberg Depression Rating Scale

The scale (Appendix B) should be used by doctors or psychologists trained in psychiatry who have sufficient clinical experience. The ten items are assessed on the basis of a clinical interview and observation. The interview should begin with more general questions and lead on to detailed symptoms. If the patient does not give exact answers, all relevant information from other sources should be integrated into the final evaluation. About 15 minutes seem to be sufficient for the interview. The rating time and length of the interview should be fixed if the scale is used to study the longitudinal course of depressive symptoms.

Each item is rated on a seven-point scale (0–6). Descriptions are given for points 0, 2, 4, and 6 on the scale as anchor points. In the analysis, the scores for each item are summed to give a total score, which can range from 0–60 points. A less expensive version of the scale, which does not include the anchor points, is available and has demonstrated validity and clinical utility [77].

The scale is especially indicated for studies on the clinical course of depression during treatment because it focuses on depression severity and does not cover a broad spectrum of depression symptoms. It is a very economical approach for such settings, given the limited number of items and short duration of the interview. The precise wording of the items guarantees good inter-rater reliability without intensive rater training. Other scales, such as the HAM-D, are preferable if a broader spectrum of symptoms needs to be covered.

Quality and characteristics of the Montgomery-Åsberg Depression Rating Scale

The original selection of items was based on the Comprehensive Psychopathological Rating Scale (CPRS) [78], which indicates the content validity. On the basis of frequency analyses and by selecting the items that showed the highest change score and correlated most strongly with the change in the total score, the original number of items related to depression was reduced to ten. The scale includes the main symptoms of depressive illness and most of the DSM criteria for depression, even though certain important areas (eg, psychomotor retardation, tendency to somatize) have been omitted as a result of the method of item selection [79].

As to other aspects of content validity, the scale correlates well with the HAM-D [6,45], especially with the first factor of the HAM-D. Meier et al [46] found a correlation between the MADRS and HAM-D-17 total scores of r=0.85 and between the MADRS and HAM-D-21 total scores of 0.83. Overall, factor analyses and correlations with the HAM-D (particularly with the various subscales) show that the MADRS covers more purely psychological symptoms than the HAM-D [6,79–86]. In these analyses, the dimensions covered by the MADRS items were classified under the headings sadness/pessimistic thoughts, inner tension, inability to feel and reduced appetite. Although the scale does not seem to be unidimensional, it should be noted that more of the MADRS items are loaded on the first factor than are the HAM-D items.

The Rasch model indicated that the MADRS seems to ensure invariance of meaning across different subgroups and also longitudinally [55,80]. As to its discriminant validity, a point of criticism is its only moderate correlation (0.42) with an anxiety scale, the Covi Anxiety Scale [46], and with different subscales of the Positive and Negative Syndrome Scale (PANSS; eg, 0.51 with the PANSS negative subscale) [87].

In the studies performed while the scale was being constructed, the sensitivity to change was claimed to be better than that of other procedures used simultaneously [88–90]. In later studies, the sensitivity of the MADRS for differences in the severity of depression [79] and change in depression symptoms was again shown to be good [80,91,92]. However, when the mean score values of the MADRS were compared with those of the HAM-D in a large sample of inpatients with major depressive disorder, the course appeared to be relatively similar, apart from the higher mean values of the MADRS [93] (Figure 2.2). The effect sizes in placebo-controlled antidepressant efficacy studies were similar to those of the HAM-D-17 scale [94] or slightly better [85,95].

Reference values are available for several clinical samples [80,81], but norm values for the general population are not, as is the case for most scales.

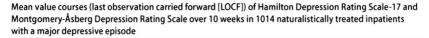

Mean value courses (last observation carried forward [LOCF]) of Hamilton Depression Rating Scale-17 and Montgomery-Åsberg Depression Rating Scale over 10 weeks in 1014 naturalistically treated inpatients with a major depressive episode

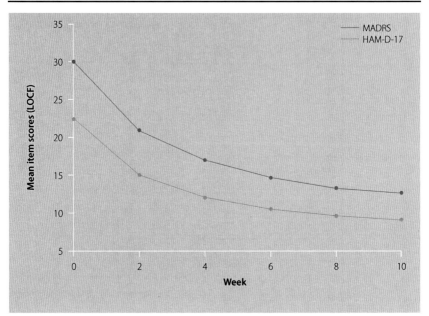

Figure 2.2 Mean value courses (last observation carried forward [LOCF]) of Hamilton Depression Rating Scale-17 and Montgomery-Åsberg Depression Rating Scale over 10 weeks in 1014 naturalistically treated inpatients with a major depressive episode. Reproduced with permission from Seemuller et al [93] ©Elsevier.

The inter-rater reliability has been presented for different samples and been shown to be high, with values of 0.89 to 0.97 [6,88]. It was found to be slightly lower in studies that included different professions (psychiatrists, psychologists, nurses) working in psychiatry [80], whereby ratings by nurses showed the lowest inter-rater reliability. The correlation with the Clinical Global Impression of Severity was approximately 0.70 in two studies [45,84]. As mentioned above, drug treatment studies in depression are increasingly using remission as a relevant categorical efficacy criterion. Various suggestions have been made for the remission cut-off score for the MADRS scale: ≤8 [96], <10 [97], or ≤10 [98].

References

1 Moller HJ. Standardised rating scales in psychiatry: methodological basis, their possibilities and limitations and descriptions of important rating scales. *World J Biol Psychiatry.* 2009;10:6-26.
2 Arbeitsgemeinschaft für Methodik und Dokumentation in der Psychiatrie. *Das AMDP-System. Manual zur Dokumentation Psychiatrischer Befunde.* 7th edn. Göttingen, Germany: Hogrefe; 2000.

3 Moller HJ, Jager M, Riedel M, Obermeier M, Strauss A, Bottlender R. The Munich 15-year follow-up study (MUFUSSAD) on first-hospitalized patients with schizophrenic or affective disorders: comparison of psychopathological and psychosocial course and outcome and prediction of chronicity. *Eur Arch Psychiatry Clin Neurosci.* 2010;260:367-384.

4 Hamilton M. A rating scale for depression. *J Neurol Neurosurg Psychiatry.* 1960;23:56-62.

5 Hamilton M. Hamilton Depression Scale. In: *ECDEU assessment manual for psychopharmacology.* Guy W, Ed. Rockville, MD: National Institute of Mental Health, 1976;193-198.

6 Montgomery SA, Asberg M. A new depression scale designed to be sensitive to change. *Br J Psychiatry.* 1979;134:382-389.

7 Goldberg DP. *The Detection of Psychiatric Illness by Questionnaire.* London: Oxford University Press; 1972.

8 Hamilton M. The assessment of anxiety states by rating. *Br J Med Psychol.* 1959;32:50-55.

9 Hamilton M. Development of a rating scale for primary depressive illness. *Br J Soc Clin Psychol.* 1967;6:278-296.

10 Posner K, Brown GK, Stanley B et al. The Columbia-Suicide Severity Rating Scale: initial validity and internal consistency findings from three multisite studies with adolescents and adults. *Am J Psychiatry.* 2011;168:1266-1277.

11 Hasemann K. Verhaltensbeobachtung. In: *Handbuch der Psychologie.* 3rd edn. Heiss R, ed. Göttingen, Germany: Hogrefe; 1971;807-836.

12 Steinmeyer EM, Moller HJ. Facet theoretic analysis of the Hamilton-D scale. *J Affect Disord.* 1992;25:53-61.

13 Bech P. Rating scales for affective disorders: their validity and consistency. *Acta Psychiatr Scand Suppl.* 1981;295:1-101.

14 Kobak KA, Greist JH, Jefferson JW et al. Computer-administered clinical rating scales. A review. *Psychopharmacology (Berl).* 1996;127:291-301.

15 Kobak KA, Greist JH, Jefferson JW et al. Computerized assessment of depression and anxiety over the telephone using interactive voice response. *MD Comput.* 1999;16:64-68.

16 Mundt JC. Interactive voice response systems in clinical research and treatment. *Psychiatr Serv.* 1997;48:611-612.

17 Bech P. Fifty years with the Hamilton scales for anxiety and depression. A tribute to Max Hamilton. *Psychother Psychosom.* 2009;78:202-211.

18 Möller HJ. Methodological aspects in the assessment of severity of depression by the Hamilton Depression Scale. *Eur Arch Psychiatry Clin Neurosci.* 2001;251(suppl 2:II):13-20.

19 Bech P. The use of rating scales in affective disorders. *European Psychiatry.* 2008;1:14-18.

20 Rush AJ, Giles DE, Schlesser MA et al. The Inventory for Depressive Symptomatology (IDS): preliminary findings. *Psychiatry Res.* 1986;18:65-87.

21 Sachs GS, Guille C, McMurrich SL. A clinical monitoring form for mood disorders. *Bipolar Disord.* 2002;4:323-327.

22 Rush AJ, Trivedi MH, Ibrahim HM et al. The 16-Item Quick Inventory of Depressive Symptomatology (QIDS), clinician rating (QIDS-C), and self-report (QIDS-SR): a psychometric evaluation in patients with chronic major depression. *Biol Psychiatry.* 2003;54:573-583.

23 Weissman MM, Sholomskas D, John K. The assessment of social adjustment. An update. *Arch Gen Psychiatry.* 1981;38:1250-1258.

24 Faltermaier T, Hecht H, Wittchen HU. *Die Social Interview Schedule (Deutschsprachige Modifizierte Version).* Regensburg, Germany: Roderer; 1987.

25 Möller HJ, Schmid-Bode W, Cording-Tommel C et al. Psychopathological and social outcome in schizophrenia versus affective/schizoaffective psychoses and prediction of poor outcome in schizophrenia. Results from a 5-8 year follow-up. *Acta Psychiatr Scand.* 1988;77:379-389.

26 Jablensky A, Schwarz R, Tomow T. WHO collaborative study on impairments and disabilities associated with schizophrenic disorders. A preliminary communication: objectives and methods. *Acta Psychiatr Scand.* 1980;62:152-159.

27 Endicott J, Spitzer RL, Fleiss JL et al. The global assessment scale. A procedure for measuring overall severity of psychiatric disturbance. *Arch Gen Psychiatry.* 1976;33:766-771.

28 Goldman HH, Skodol AE, Lave TR. Revising axis V for DSM-IV: a review of measures of social functioning. *Am J Psychiatry*. 1992;149:1148-1156.

29 Morosini PL, Magliano L, Brambilla L et al. Development, reliability and acceptability of a new version of the DSM-IV Social and Occupational Functioning Assessment Scale (SOFAS) to assess routine social functioning. *Acta Psychiatr Scand*. 2000;101:323-329.

30 Bottlender R, Strauss A, Moller HJ. Social disability in schizophrenic, schizoaffective and affective disorders 15 years after first admission. *Schizophr Res*. 2010;116:9-15.

31 Bech P, Coppen A. *The Hamilton Scales*. Psychopharmacology Series 9. Berlin: Springer-Verlag; 1990.

32 Gibbons RD, Clark DC, Kupfer DJ. Exactly what does the Hamilton Depression Rating Scale measure? *J Psychiatr Res*. 1993;27:259-273.

33 Bech P. *Clinical Psychometrics*. 1st edn. Chichester, UK: Wiley-Blackwell; 2012.

34 Collegium Internationale Psychiatriae Scalarum (CIPS). *Rating Scales for Psychiatry*. 5th edn. Weinheim, Germany: Beltz; 1990.

35 Moller HJ, Glaser K, Leverkus F, et al. Double-blind, multicenter comparative study of sertraline versus amitriptyline in outpatients with major depression. *Pharmacopsychiatry*. 2000;33:206-212.

36 Moller HJ, Volz HP, Reimann IW et al. Opipramol for the treatment of generalized anxiety disorder: a placebo-controlled trial including an alprazolam-treated group. *J Clin Psychopharmacol*. 2001;21:59-65.

37 Moller HJ. Scales used in depression and anxiety research. In: *Handbook of Depression and Anxiety*. Kasper S, den Boer JA, Sitsen JM, eds. New York, Basel: Marcel Decker; 2003:789-808.

38 Baumann U. [Methodologic studies of the Hamilton rating scale for depression (author's transl)]. *Arch Psychiatr Nervenkr*. 1976;222:359-375.

39 Cicchetti DV, Prusoff BA. Reliability of depression and associated clinical symptoms. *Arch Gen Psychiatry*. 1983;40:987-990.

40 Waldron J, Bates TJ. The management of depression in hospital. A comparative trial of desipramine and Imipramine. *Br J Psychiatry*. 1965;111:511-516.

41 Williams JB. A structured interview guide for the Hamilton Depression Rating Scale. *Arch Gen Psychiatry*. 1988;45:742-747.

42 Bech P, Kastrup M, Rafaelsen OJ. Mini-compendium of rating scales for states of anxiety depression mania schizophrenia with corresponding DSM-III syndromes. *Acta Psychiatr Scand Suppl*. 1986;326:1-37.

43 Hedlund JL. The Hamilton Rating Scale for Depression : A comprehensive review. *J Operational Psychiatry*. 1979;10:149-165.

44 Maier W, Philipp M, Heuser I et al. Improving depression severity assessment--I. Reliability, internal validity and sensitivity to change of three observer depression scales. *J Psychiatr Res*. 1988;22:3-12.

45 Welner J. Eine internationale multizentrische Doppelblind-Prüfung eines neuen Antidepressivums. In: *Depressive Zustände*. Kielholz P, ed. Vienna: Huber; 1972.

46 Maier W, Heuser I, Philipp M, et al. Improving depression severity assessment--II. Content, concurrent and external validity of three observer depression scales. *J Psychiatr Res*. 1988;22:13-19.

47 Moller HJ. Rating depressed patients: observer- vs self-assessment. *Eur Psychiatry*. 2000;15:160-172.

48 Montgomery SA, Kasper S. Severe depression and antidepressants: focus on a pooled analysis of placebo-controlled studies on agomelatine. *Int Clin Psychopharmacol*. 2007;22:283-291.

49 Cuijpers P, van Straten A, Warmerdam L, et al. Psychotherapy versus the combination of psychotherapy and pharmacotherapy in the treatment of depression: a meta-analysis. *Depress Anxiety*. 2009;26:279-288.

50 Khan A, Faucett J, Lichtenberg P, et al. A systematic review of comparative efficacy of treatments and controls for depression. *PLoS One*. 2012;7:e41778.

51 Zimmerman M, Chelminski I, Posternak M. A review of studies of the Hamilton depression rating scale in healthy controls: implications for the definition of remission in treatment studies of depression. *J Nerv Ment Dis*. 2004;192:595-601.

52 Bech P, Fava M, Trivedi MH, et al. Factor structure and dimensionality of the two depression scales in STAR*D using level 1 datasets. *J Affect Disord*. 2011;132:396-400.

53 Rush AJ, Gullion CM, Basco MR, et al. The Inventory of Depressive Symptomatology (IDS): psychometric properties. *Psychol Med*. 1996;26:477-486.

54 Maier W, Philipp M, Gerken A. [Dimensions of the Hamilton Depression Scale. Factor analysis studies]. *Eur Arch Psychiatry Neurol Sci.* 1985; 234:417-422.

55 Bech P, Gram LF, Dein E, et al. Quantitative rating of depressive states. *Acta Psychiatr Scand.* 1975; 51:161-170.

56 Maier W, Philipp M. Improving the assessment of severity of depressive states: a reduction of the Hamilton Depression Scale. *Pharmacopsychiatry.* 1985;18:114-115.

57 McIntyre R, Kennedy S, Bagby RM, et al. Assessing full remission. *J Psychiatry Neurosci.* 2002;27:235-239.

58 McIntyre RS, Konarski JZ, Mancini DA, et al. Measuring the severity of depression and remission in primary care: validation of the HAM-D-7 scale. *CMAJ.* 2005;173:1327-1334.

59 Bech P. Meta-analysis of placebo-controlled trials with mirtazapine using the core items of the Hamilton Depression Scale as evidence of a pure antidepressive effect in the short-term treatment of major depression. *Int J Neuropsychopharmacol.* 2001; 4:337-345.

60 Ballesteros J, Bobes J, Bulbena A et al. Sensitivity to change, discriminative performance, and cutoff criteria to define remission for embedded short scales of the Hamilton depression rating scale (HAM-D). *J Affect Disord.* 2007;102:93-99.

61 Ruhe HG, Dekker JJ, Peen J, et al. Clinical use of the Hamilton Depression Rating Scale: is increased efficiency possible? A post hoc comparison of Hamilton Depression Rating Scale, Maier and Bech subscales, Clinical Global Impression, and Symptom Checklist-90 scores. *Compr Psychiatry.* 2005;46:417-427.

62 Faries D, Herrera J, Rayamajhi J et al. The responsiveness of the Hamilton Depression Rating Scale. *J Psychiatr Res.* 2000;34:3-10.

63 Entsuah R, Shaffer M, Zhang J. A critical examination of the sensitivity of unidimensional subscales derived from the Hamilton Depression Rating Scale to antidepressant drug effects. *J Psychiatr Res.* 2002;36:437-448.

64 Bech P. The instrumental use of rating scales for depression. *Pharmacopsychiatry.* 1984;17:22-28.

65 Carroll BJ, Feinberg M, Smouse PE et al. The Carroll rating scale for depression. I. Development, reliability and validation. *Br J Psychiatry.* 1981;138:194-200.

66 Reynolds WM, Kobak KA. Development and validation of the Hamilton Depression Inventory: A self-report version of the Hamilton Depression Rating Scale. *Psychological Assessment.* 1995;7:472-83.

67 Kobak KA, Reynolds WM, Rosenfeld R, et al. Development and validation of a computer-administered Hamilton Depression Rating Scale. *Psychological Assessment.* 1990;2:56-63.

68 Kobak KA, Mundt JC, Greist JH, et al. Computer assessment of depression: Automating the Hamilton Depression Rating Scale. *Drug Inf J.* 2000;34:145-156.

69 Bent-Hansen J, Bech P. Validity of the definite and semidefinite questionnaire version of the Hamilton Depression Scale, the Hamilton Subscale and the Melancholia Scale. Part I. *Eur Arch Psychiatry Clin Neurosci.* 2011;261:37-46.

70 Frank E, Prien RF, Jarrett RB, et al. Conceptualization and rationale for consensus definitions of terms in major depressive disorder. Remission, recovery, relapse, and recurrence. *Arch Gen Psychiatry.* 1991;48:851-855.

71 Rush AJ, Kraemer HC, Sackeim HA, et al. Report by the ACNP Task Force on response and remission in major depressive disorder. *Neuropsychopharmacology.* 2006;31:1841-1853.

72 Moller HJ. Outcomes in major depressive disorder: the evolving concept of remission and its implications for treatment. *World J Biol Psychiatry.* 2008;9:102-114.

73 Zimmerman M, Posternak MA, Chelminski I. Heterogeneity among depressed outpatients considered to be in remission. *Compr Psychiatry.* 2007;48:113-117.

74 Zimmerman M, Posternak MA, Ruggero CJ. Impact of study design on the results of continuation studies of antidepressants. *J Clin Psychopharmacol.* 2007;27:177-181.

75 Zimmerman M, Posternak MA, Chelminski I. Defining remission on the Montgomery-Åsberg depression rating scale. *J Clin Psychiatry.* 2004;65:163-168.

76 Zimmerman M, Posternak MA, Chelminski I. Is the cutoff to define remission on the Hamilton Rating Scale for Depression too high? *J Nerv Ment Dis.* 2005;193:170-175.

77 Moller HJ, Schnitker J. [Prospective study using a modified Montgomery-Åsberg Depression Scale]. *Nervenarzt.* 2007;78:685-690.

78 Asberg M, Montgomery SA, Perris C et al. A comprehensive psychopathological rating scale. *Acta Psychiatr Scand Suppl.* 1978:5-27.

79 Kearns NP, Cruickshank CA, McGuigan KJ et al. A comparison of depression rating scales. *Br J Psychiatry.* 1982;141:45-49.

80 Schmidtke A, Fleckenstein P, Moises W et al. [Studies of the reliability and validity of the German version of the Montgomery-Asberg Depression Rating Scale (MADRS)]. *Schweiz Arch Neurol Psychiatr.* 1988;139:51-65.

81 Maier W, Philipp M. Comparative analysis of observer depression scales. *Acta Psychiatr Scand.* 1985;72:239-245.

82 Craighead WE, Evans DD. Factor analysis of the Montgomery-Asberg Depression Rating Scale. *Depression.* 1996; 4:31-33.

83 Hammond MF. Rating depression severity in the elderly physically ill patient: reliability and factor structure of the Hamilton and the Montgomery-Asberg Depression Rating Scales. *Int J Geriatr Psychiatry.* 1998;13:257-261.

84 Neumann NU, Schulte RM. Montgomery-Åsberg-Depressions-Rating-Skala Bestimmung der Validität und Interrater-Reliabilität der deutschen Fassung. *Psycho.* 1989;14:911-924.

85 Bech P, Tanghoj P, Andersen HF et al. Citalopram dose-response revisited using an alternative psychometric approach to evaluate clinical effects of four fixed citalopram doses compared to placebo in patients with major depression. *Psychopharmacology (Berl).* 2002;163:20-25.

86 Mokken RJ. *A theory and procedure of scale analysis with applications in political research. Methods and models in the social sciences, 1.* The Hague, Netherlands: Mouton; 1971.

87 Wolthaus JE, Dingemans PM, Schene AH, et al. Component structure of the positive and negative syndrome scale (PANSS) in patients with recent-onset schizophrenia and spectrum disorders. *Psychopharmacology (Berl).* 2000;150:399-403.

88 Montgomery S, Asberg M, Jornestedt L et al. Reliability of the CPRS between the disciplines of psychiatry, general practice, nursing and psychology in depressed patients. *Acta Psychiatr Scand Suppl.* 1978:29-32.

89 Montgomery SA, Montgomery DB. Measurement of change in psychiatric illness: new obsessional, schizophrenia and depression scales. *Postgrad Med J.* 1980; 56(Suppl 1):50-52.

90 Montgomery SA, Smeyatsky N, de Ruiter M, et al. Profiles of antidepressant activity with the Montgomery-Asberg Depression Rating Scale. *Acta Psychiatr Scand Suppl.* 1985;320:38-42.

91 Deloch E. Vortrag auf dem Idom-Expertengespräch in Estoril. *G Selecta Bericht.* 1986;42:3068-3070.

92 Gutzmann H. Vortrag auf dem Idom-Expertengespräch in Estoril. *G Selecta Bericht.* 1986;42:3068-3070.

93 Seemuller F, Riedel M, Obermeier M, et al. Outcomes of 1014 naturalistically treated inpatients with major depressive episode. *Eur Neuropsychopharmacol.* 2010;20:346-55.

94 Khan A, Khan SR, Shankles EB, et al. Relative sensitivity of the Montgomery-Asberg Depression Rating Scale, the Hamilton Depression rating scale and the Clinical Global Impressions rating scale in antidepressant clinical trials. *Int Clin Psychopharmacol.* 2002;17:281-285.

95 Calabrese JR, Bowden CL, Sachs GS et al. A double-blind placebo-controlled study of lamotrigine monotherapy in outpatients with bipolar I depression. Lamictal 602 Study Group. *J Clin Psychiatry.* 1999;60:79-88.

96 Carmody TJ, Rush AJ, Bernstein I, et al. The Montgomery-Asberg and the Hamilton ratings of depression: a comparison of measures. *Eur Neuropsychopharmacol.* 2006;16:601-611.

97 Hawley CJ, Gale TM, Sivakumaran T. Defining remission by cut off score on the MADRS: selecting the optimal value. *J Affect Disord.* 2002;72:177-184.

98 Zimmerman M, Posternak MA, Chelminski I. Derivation of a definition of remission on the Montgomery-Asberg depression rating scale corresponding to the definition of remission on the Hamilton rating scale for depression. *J Psychiatr Res.* 2004;38:577-582.

3. Self-rating scales

Hans-Jürgen Möller

General aspects of self-rating scales

Patients use self-rating instruments to describe past or current behavior and experiences [1-4]. Self-rated scales are a cost-effective way for the doctor or researcher to obtain information about a patient's mental state and eliminate observer bias. However, like observer ratings (see Chapter 2), self-rating scales can also be distorted, although for different reasons which will be discussed later in this chapter. Generally, self-ratings are more subjective; however, observer ratings are also not fully objective. The main disadvantages of self-rating scales are as follows:

- conscious or unconscious tendencies might falsify responses (eg, tendencies to exaggerate or conceal symptoms); and
- positive response bias and social desirability effects.

These disadvantages can seriously affect the findings of self-rating instruments. Several factors might be involved, such as personality traits; for example, higher neuroticism generally leads to higher scores on self-rating depression scales or related complaints lists [5]. Also, the severity of the mental disorder can affect results. For example, severely depressed patients often underestimate the severity of their depression, while mildly depressed patients overestimate it [5]. The latter case may have consequences in a treatment study, for example when the participants' mental condition appears to improve over the course of treatment if scales are used as the determinant. Such tendencies are only partially detectable through the use of control scales, which are commonly used, especially in personality tests (which are based on self-ratings).

Another disadvantage of self-rating scales is that they usually have a higher variance than observer rating scales. Consequently, if self-rating instruments are used, sample sizes need to be larger in order for the study to achieve statistical significance. At present, drug authorities do not accept the results of self-rating scales as the only outcome measurement in drug studies for several reasons, including those mentioned above.

© Springer International Publishing Switzerland 2014
G. Alexopoulos et al., *Guide to Assessment Scales in Major Depressive Disorder*,
DOI 10.1007/978-3-319-04627-3_3

Because of all these limitations, a careful decision needs to be made whether or not to use a self-rating scale for depression and whether the scale will be used alone or with an observer rating scale. A self-rating might be sufficiently valid as a screening test for depression (eg, the Major Depression Inventory [MDI] questionnaire [1,6], which is based on the MDI observer rating, or the depression-related part of the Patient Health Questionnaire [PHQ-9] [7], or even quite short self-ratings that do not directly focus on the concept of depression but rather on well-being, such as the World Health Organization [WHO]-Five Well-being Index [1]). A self-rating scale may also be used to measure treatment effects in depression, as was done for example in the North American Sequenced Treatment Alternatives to Relieve Depression (STAR*D) study [8], to evaluate the severity of depression cross-sectionally or the course of depression longitudinally during routine patient care. However, for more sophisticated research studies, especially clinical studies for regulatory approval of an antidepressant, it is advisable to combine a self-rating scale with an observer rating.

Symptom assessment

Self-assessment procedures are available for assessing the symptoms and syndromes of depression; examples include the Beck Depression Inventory (BDI) [9] for depressive symptoms and the Clinical Self-Rating Scales (CSRS) [10–14] and Symptom Checklist-90 (SCL-90), which will be discussed later in the chapter, for depressive, somatic, and paranoid symptoms [15]. Self-rated scales can also be in the form of visual analogue scales (so-called 'barometer scales' on which particular dimensions or current experience are graphically represented); these are especially useful for intra-individual studies of course over time with a multitude of sequential measurement points [16,17].

Apart from a few scales that measure a broad spectrum of subjectively experienced alterations in the current mental state (eg, SCL-90), most self-rated scales focus on specific aspects of disturbance of subjective experience. Examples are depressive symptom scales [13,18,19], anxiety symptoms scales [20,21] and measures of current mood or subjective well-being [1,11]. One of the advantages of this approach is that the quantity of items is limited, a particular strength when severely disturbed psychiatric patients are being evaluated.

In order to obtain a sufficiently clear subjective view of the current psychological state, it is always preferable to present not only a checklist of adjectives describing complaints, but also a symptom-oriented scale (eg, Self-Rating Depression Scale [SRDS]) [19], which is more closely linked to the symptom-oriented, observer rating approach. However, a precise differentiation between different aspects of the 'subjective state' is generally not useful compared to the detailed measurement of psychological disturbances by observer evaluation [22]. In fact, when results from clinical self-rating scales are compared with those of observer-rated scales administered by specialists, the various dimensions of the subjective state described by self-rated instruments seem to be more similar to one another than to the different aspects of psychopathology delineated by clinical observer-rated assessments.

This finding was supported by a joint factor analysis of data from observer ratings and self-ratings of mental states [23]. This study applied the Inpatient Multidimensional Psychiatric Scale (IMPS) [24] as an observer-rated measure and the CSRS [10–14] as a self-rating measure. The self-assessed data were mainly represented in a single factor (the first to emerge) while the observer-rated data were distributed across five further factors. However, this secondary factor analysis (in which the primary factors derived from the initial analysis of each scale were also entered as variables) does not demonstrate that self-assessment simply produces a factor reflecting a global 'tendency to complain' rather than a differentiated picture of subjective impairment. Primary factor analysis of single items from the CSRS and other self-rating instruments indicates that different dimensions of disturbances, such as depressiveness, paranoid tendencies and somatic complaints, certainly can be differentiated on a subjective level. However, the depressiveness factor is closely associated with the various other types of subjective disturbance. In this context, it should be mentioned that psychotic symptoms assessed with the SCl-90 seem to be closely correlated with depressive symptoms and apparently have another meaning than observer-rated psychotic symptoms, with which they are not closely correlated [25]. A further consideration is that the correlations between the different dimensions and between their change scores are very high (Möller; unpublished data), so that the specificity of each of these self-rated dimensions should not be overinterpreted.

The level of agreement between self-assessment and observer assessment varies and depends on the type of disturbance and symptom severity [2,26–31]. For example, when depressive symptomatology is severe, as at the time of inpatient admission, the concordance is substantially lower than after partial remission of symptoms. This finding is probably associated with the more limited capacity for self-observation among the severely depressed and also with the fact that observers tend to identify very severe depressive symptoms to a greater extent on the basis of non-verbal evidence than they do less severe depressive symptoms, for which the patients' verbal reports are more important. Patients with dysthymia ('neurotic depression') show a greater tendency than patients with endogenous depression to overstate their symptoms.

The type of the rating scale (symptom list or adjective scale) and the item selection are of great importance for the correlation between self-ratings and observer ratings of depressive symptomatology. One might assume that the best correlation would be obtained if the selection and wording of the items in the self-rating scale correspond more or less fully with those in the observer rating scale. However, patients may have difficulty understanding a direct 'translation' of an observer scale into a self-rating version. Some studies on correlations between self-rating and observer ratings have been performed. For example, the SRDS [19] correlates only moderately with the Hamilton Depression Rating Scale (HAM-D; r=0.41) [32], as does the BDI [33] with the self-rating version of the Inventory of Depressive Symptomatology

(IDS-SR) [34]. In contrast, the correlation between the Carroll self-rating version of the HAM-D (CRS) [35] and the observer rated HAM-D was 0.80. Rush et al reported interestingly high correlations between the more or less identical observer rating and self-rating versions of the IDS and between each of them and the HAM-D [36,37]. The degree of concordance between self-rating and observer rating scales is substantially greater for the amount of change over time, as measured in longitudinal studies, than when psychopathological phenomena are recorded at a single point in time [14,38].

It seems plausible that scales with similar items on both self-rating and observer rating scales might have a higher degree of concordance than an observer-rated symptom scale like the HAM-D and an adjective mood scale for self-rating, for example. However, because of the factors mentioned above and a possibly different interpretation of the symptom descriptions by doctors and patients, and especially because patients usually do not perceive alterations in, for example, their mimic and motor behavior (which is an important way for doctors to assess depression), concordance can still be limited even if the symptom selection is similar. This can lead to relevant differences in score and in categories that depend on the score values (eg, response or remission criteria) [26,31,39]. This was evident in a study by Rush et al [37] that compared the percentages of remitters in an antidepressant study by using the IDS-SR-30 and 16-Item Quick Inventory of Depressive Symptomology (QIDS-SR-16) self-rating scales and the

Differences between depressive self-rating and observer rating scales in determining remission

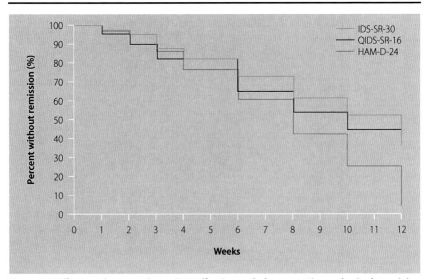

Figure 3.1 Differences between depressive self-rating and observer rating scales in determining remission. Time to remission as determined by total score at exit for 30-item Inventory of Depressive Symptomatology, Self-Report [IDS-SR30] (≤14), 16-item Quick Inventory of Depressive Symptomatology, Self-Report [QIDS-SR-16] (≤6) and 24-item Hamilton Rating Scale for Depression [HAM-D24] (≤8). Reproduced with permission from Möller et al [38] ©Karger.

HAM-D-24 (Figure 3.1). The difference in remission rates between the two self-rating scales was relatively low, while the difference in remission rates between the two self-rating scales and the HAM-D-24 was high and, despite being quite similar to the self-rating results in the first 5 weeks, increased from the sixth to the twelfth week. The results of the first treatment phase of the STAR*D study are also of interest in this context: while the self-rating with QIDS identified 32% remitters, the HAM-D identified only 27% [8].

As previously mentioned, a combination of self-rated and observer rated scales is the best approach to ensure that both subjective and objective psychopathological states are described in a complementary way. Measures of subjective well-being are of particular interest for treatment assessments with short rating intervals, particularly visual analogue scales (sometimes called barometer scales) and adjective mood scales. These scales measure current disturbances of mood and lend themselves especially well to repeated measurements. Measures of well-being allow a very good description of response to a therapeutic intervention at the self-assessment level. Modern methods of statistical analysis, such as some of the procedures developed for time series analysis, allow satisfactory analysis of such data [40,41].

Examples of self-rating scales in depression

Several self-rating scales for depression are available either as symptom lists or adjective mood lists. In contrast to the situation with the observer rating scales for depression, where two scales are predominantly used (HAM-D and Montgomery-Åsberg Depression Scale), no single self-rating scale is recommended above the others. A possible explanation for this might be that self-rating scales are used in more varied situations than observer ratings and different self-rating approaches are meaningful, depending on the respective indication. For example, for a simple screening, scales such as the PHQ-9 (the depression score), the self-rating version of the MDI, or even the short WHO-5 Well-being Index might be sufficient. For frequent repetition of treatment effects in short intervals (eg, daily or even several times a day), an adjective mood list or barometer scale is optimal, especially when combined with an observer rating depression score applied at longer intervals (for example, each week) to increase the validity of the simple self-rating scale being used. For the cross-sectional assessment of depression severity and documentation of the course of depression under treatment conditions, a more detailed self-rating scale like the Beck Depression Inventory (BDI) [18,42] or a self-rating version of the HAM-D [35] might be the best among the self-rating options. The BDI is used in most psychotherapy studies, especially those on cognitive behavior therapy.

Zung Self-Rating Depression Scale
The Self-Rating Depression Scale (SDS) was developed by Zung [19] in analogy to his observer rated depression scale, the Depression Status Inventory [43]. Although the SDS has proven clinical value, it is no longer widely used. The self-rating scale consists of 20 items covering

typical symptoms, experiences and complaints of depressed patients. The frequencies of the phenomena in the past 7 days are rated on a four-point scale that ranges from 1 (never) to 4 (mostly/always). The sum of the item scores builds the total score. The scale is valid to describe the cross-sectional severity of depression or, if sequentially applied, the change in severity.

The scale has content validity because of the selection of items, which are characteristic for depressed patients. Moderate correlations were found with the HAM-D [44], but, as to be expected, higher correlations (0.70) were found with the self-rated depression scale of the Minnesota Multiphasic Personality Inventory [45].

Hospital Anxiety and Depression Scale

The Hospital Anxiety and Depression Scale (HADS) was developed by Zigmond and Snaith [46], mainly for use in patients with depression suffering from a somatic illness (Appendix C). However, the scale can also be used to assess short- and long-term severity of depression. The primary intention of the HADS is to focus on the assessment of depression and anxiety in patients in nonpsychiatric medical institutions, who usually show fewer or less severe mental disturbances and non-specific symptoms. Depression and anxiety were selected for the scale because they are the most prevalent mental symptoms in this patient population and are often difficult to differentiate.

The HADS consists of 14 items related to depression (7 items) and anxiety (7 items); items are rated on a four-point scale (0–3). The items were selected from the Clinical Anxiety Scale [47] and the Present State Examination [48]. The depression items are mostly related to anhedonia, which is considered to be a central aspect of depression. The items are evaluated regarding frequency or intensity and pre-post change or planned/actual comparison. The item scores are summed to give either a depression score or an anxiety score (maximum score of 21 for each). Occasionally, a total score is also calculated and interpreted as 'mental distress'. During the rating, which takes about 2–6 minutes, the patients evaluate their symptoms and experiences in the past week. The terms anxiety and depression are not mentioned in the scale and should also not be mentioned by the respective investigator. If necessary, the items can be read aloud by an investigator, who then documents the patient's responses.

The psychometric properties are reported in the review by Bjelland et al [49]. The interrater reliability over several weeks is in the range of approximately 0.70–0.80, as is to be expected for slowly changing mood alterations. The content validity is primarily given through the item selection. However, the depression concept underlying item selection is more limited than both the traditional clinical concept of depression and the traditional depression scales and is, therefore, more relevant for a population with minor changes. As for convergent validity, Zigmond and Snaith reported correlations of 0.54 with anxiety observer ratings and 0.74 with depression observer ratings [46]. Correlations with respective self-ratings or observer ratings were also described in later studies [50]. Results regarding discriminant validity are extremely inconsistent. The original publication from Zigmond and Snaith [46] described very positive validity results, probably because the authors focused on the correlation with the respective observer rated dimensions. However, a later study focusing on correlations with the (self-rated) State Trait Anxiety Inventory (STAI) found that the STAI correlated to a similar degree with both the anxiety and the depression subscale of the HADS (approximately 0.60 for both) [51,52].

As to sensitivity to change, only a few medication studies have been performed [53,54], but several psychosocial studies in patients suffering from cancer or heart disease (see [50]). Factor analytical studies suggest a two-factor structure with 50–70% of explained variance [49,50,55]. However, the intercorrelation between the two subscores is moderate to high (approximately 0.40 to 0.70), indicating the close relationship between depressive and anxiety symptoms [56]. Norms of a representative sample of the general population, as well as reference values for several clinical samples, are available [57].

90-Item Self-Report Symptom Inventory

The SCL-90 is the revised version of the Hopkins Symptom Check List [15,58–60]. The scale is used for patients to assess various burdening symptoms. It allows nine ranges of syndromes to be recorded and was specifically constructed to register the effects of drug treatment. It has been used in various clinical studies with neuroleptics, tranquilizers and antidepressants [61,62].

Paranoid Depression Scale

The Paranoid Depression Scale [PDS], which is available in two parallel forms, is composed of 43 items [10–14,63]. It records the degree of subjective impairment resulting from emotional reduction due to anxious-depressive mood (these items are also on a separate depression scale) and a distinct cognitive dimension to determine a distrusting attitude and whether the subject is out of touch with reality. In addition, the scale includes eight control items that measure disease denial and three items that assess motivation. The values of the individual items are summarized as factor values.

Indicators of the validity include correlations of the paranoid scale with the criterion of belonging to a group of schizophrenic patients, correlations of the depression scale with the criterion of belonging to a group of patients with depressive mood, correlations with relevant factors of other scales and sensitivity in the recording of therapy-induced changes. The depression scale is also available as a separate, 16-item scale that does not include the items of the paranoid scale. Norm values are available for a representative sample of the general population in Germany and reference values are available for various clinical groups (physically ill, mixed psychiatric groups, individual psychiatric diagnosis groups).

Adjective Mood Scale

The Adjective Mood Scale (AMS) contains 28 items and is available in two parallel versions [10–14,63]. It records the degree of current alterations of subjective well-being. The scale is especially indicated for mood course descriptions with a focus on fast mood alterations. For this reason the test can be frequently repeated. It is suitable for healthy subjects and physically or mentally ill patients, particularly mentally ill patients with affective disorders. The values of the individual items are summed to give a total score, which indicates the impairment in subjective well-being. High inter- and intraindividual correlations with global assessments of depressive mood and the sensitivity for recording therapy-induced changes prove the validity. Norm values are available for a representative sample of the general population of the former West Germany and reference values are available for various clinical groups.

Featured scale: Beck Depression Inventory

The BDI is a frequently used self-rating scale that was originally developed as an observer rating scale and further developed into a self-rating instrument shortly thereafter [18,42]. Certain aspects of the scale were then revised to avoid ambiguities in the item formulation, among other things; a revised version was published in 1987 [64]. The BDI has 21 items and places a special focus on cognitive aspects of depression; it does not include motor or anxiety-related items. Internationally, the scale is seen as the standard self-rating scale for depression in psychotherapy studies [65], perhaps because of its focus on cognitive symptoms, but it is sometimes also used in antidepressant studies [66]. It is available in several languages and also as short versions with 13 or 6 items [67–71]. A North American version of the BDI, the BDI-II, was adapted to the Diagnostic and Statistical Manual of Mental Disorders (DSM)-IV [64].

How to use the Beck Depression Inventory
The items of the scale were selected on the basis of experience with the symptoms of depressed patients, mostly psychotherapy patients, without considering etiological aspects or diagnostic systems. The scale covers a broad spectrum of depressive symptoms, especially those related to mood and cognition.

The scale is completed by the patient and assesses depressive symptoms and the severity of depression, but does not assign symptoms to diagnostic categories [2,64,68]. The 21 items are rated on a four-point scale ranging from 0 (symptom is not present) to 3 (symptom is severe). Patients choose the level that best describes their condition in the past week (or two weeks in BDI-II) before the rating, including the day of the rating. For most of the items, patients are asked to compare their current state to a former one and to rate how much the item has improved or worsened. For most of the other items the cross-sectional degree of intensity has to be assessed directly. The total score can range from 0 to 63. Subscales can be used in addition to the total score to answer special research questions, for example a cognitive-affective or somatovegetative subscale. Such subscales are composed either on the basis of clinical considerations or by using a Rasch analysis approach to identify homogenous item groups.

Patients usually need 10–20 minutes to perform the self-rating. Besides the typical self-rating procedure, it is possible for the investigator to read the items out loud and record the patient's answers. When using this approach, one has to be careful that the investigator does not introduce any bias. To analyze the inventory, all item scores are summed up to a total score. In case of double crosses for individual items, always the highest score should be considered.

Quality and characteristics of the Beck Depression Inventory

The reliability and validity of the BDI are satisfactory [68,72,73]. The convergent validity with other self-rating scales is also relatively good; for example, the correlation with the Zung SDS is 0.72 [74]. The correlation with the observer rated HAM-D is lower (approximately 0.30 to 0.40; [75]), as would be expected, although some North American studies found higher correlation values [72]. As to discriminant validity, the scale's moderate correlations with anxiety scales are a point of criticism. However, the correlations between observer- and self-rated anxiety scales are always lower than between observer- and self-rated depression scores [76]. Furthermore, other self-rating depression scales and even observer rating scales for depression or anxiety also have problems with discriminant validity. The sensitivity for treatment-induced changes was demonstrated in several studies (see the meta-analysis by Cuijpers et al [64]).

Factorial analyses have consistently found that a 'general factor' exists, with loadings primarily on the cognitive items. Two- to seven-factor solutions were described without showing much concordance. A facet analysis described three core items: sadness, dissatisfaction and irritability; the analysis indicated that most of the other items can be considered as additive ingredients to these core items, while vegetative symptoms play only a marginal role [76]. Reference values for different clinical groups are available, but norms from a representative population are not.

References

1   Bech P. *Clinical Psychometrics*. 1st edn. Chichester, UK: Wiley-Blackwell; 2012.
2   Möller HJ. Rating depressed patients: observer- vs self-assessment. *Eur Psychiatry*. 2000;15:160-172.
3   Möller HJ. Scales ued in depression and anxiety research. In: Kasper S, den Boer JA, Sitsen JM, eds. *Handbook of Depression and Anxiety*. New York, Basel: Marcel Decker; 2003:789-808.
4   Möller HJ. Standardised rating scales in psychiatry: methodological basis, their possibilities and limitations and descriptions of important rating scales. *World J Biol Psychiatry*. 2009;10:6-26.
5   Paykel ES, Norton KRW. Self-report and clinical interview in the assessment of depression. In: Sartorius N, Ban TA , eds. *Assessment of Depression*. Heidelberg: Springer-Verlag; 1986;356-366.
6   Olsen LR, Jensen DV, Noerholm V, Martiny K, Bech P. The internal and external validity of the Major Depression Inventory in measuring severity of depressive states. *Psychol Med*. 2003;33:351-356.
7   Kroenke K, Spitzer RL, Williams JB. The PHQ-9: validity of a brief depression severity measure. *J Gen Intern Med*. 2001;16:606-613.
8   Trivedi MH, Rush AJ, Wisniewski SR, et al; for the STAR*D Study Team. Evaluation of outcomes with citalopram for depression using measurement-based care in STAR*D: implications for clinical practice. *Am J Psychiatry*. 2006;163:28-40.
9   Beck AT, Rush AJ, Shaw BF, et al. *Kognitive Therapie der Depression*. 2nd edn. Munich: Psychologie Verlags Union; 1986.
10 von Zerssen D. Klinische Selbstbeurteilungs-Skalen (KSbS) aus dem Münchener Psychiatrischen Informationssystem (PSYCHIS München). Algemeiner Teil. Weinheim: Beltz; 1976.

11 von Zerssen D. Klinische Selbstbeurteilungs-Skalen (KSbS) aus dem Münchener Psychiatrischen Informationssystem (PSYCHIS München). Befindlichkeits-Skala. Weinheim: Beltz; 1976.

12 von Zerssen D. Klinische Selbstbeurteilungs-Skalen (KSbS) aus dem Münchener Psychiatrischen Informationssystem (PSYCHIS München). Beschwerden-Liste. Weinheim: Beltz; 1976.

13 von Zerssen D. Klinische Selbstbeurteilungs-Skalen (KSbS) aus dem Münchener Psychiatrischen Informationssystem (PSYCHIS München). Paranoid-Depressivitäts-Skalen. Weinheim: Beltz; 1976.

14 von Zerssen D. Clinical Self-Rating Scaes (CSRS) of the Munich Psychiatric Information System (PSYCHIS). In: Sartorius N, Ban TA, eds. *Assessment of Depression*. Berlin: Springer; 1986:270-303.

15 Derogatis LR. SCL-90. Administration, scoring and procedures. *Manual-I for the R(evised) version and other instruments of the psychopathology rating scale series*. Baltimore, MA: Johns Hopkins University School of Medicine;1977.

16 Luria RE. The validity and reliability of the visual analogue mood scale. *J Psychiatr Res*. 1975;12:51-57.

17 Möller HJ, Blank R, Steinmeyer EM. Single-case evaluation of sleep-deprivation effects by means of nonparametric time-series analysis (according to the HTAKA model). *Eur Arch Psychiatry Neurol Sci*. 1989;239:133-139.

18 Beck AT, Ward CH, Mendelson M, Mock J, Erbaugh J. An inventory for measuring depression. *Arch Gen Psychiatry*. 1961;4:561-571.

19 Zung WW. A self-rating depression scale. *Arch Gen Psychiatry*. 1965;12:63-70.

20 Spielberg CD. *Manual for the State-Trait Anxiety Inventory (Form X-I)*. Palo Alto, CA: Consulting Psychologists Press; 1983.

21 Zung WW. A rating instrument for anxiety disorders. *Psychosomatics*. 1971;12:371-379.

22 von Zerssen D. Klinisch-psychiatrische Selbstbeurteilungs-Fragebögen. In: Baumann U, Berbalk H, Seidenstücker G, eds. *Klinische Psychologie*. Trends in Forschung und Praxis, vol 2. Bern: Huber, 1979;130-159.

23 von Zerssen D, Cording C. The measurement of change in endogenous affective disorders. *Arch Psychiatr Nervenkr*. 1978;226:95-112.

24 Lorr M. Assessing psychotic behaviour by the IMPS. In: Pichot P, Olivier-Martin R, eds. *Psychological Measurements in Psychopharmacology*. Basel: Karger; 1974:50-63.

25 Seemuller F, Riedel M, Obermeier M, et al. The validity of self-rated psychotic symptoms in depressed inpatients. *Eur Psychiatry*. 2012;27:547-552.

26 Bailey J, Coppen A. A comparison between the Hamilton Rating Scale and the Beck Inventory in the measurement of depression. *Br J Psychiatry*. 1976;128:486-489.

27 Möller HJ. Outcome criteria in antidepressant drug trials: self-rating versus observer rating scales. *Pharmacopsychiatry*. 1991;24:71-75.

28 Prusoff BA, Klerman GL, Paykel ES. Concordance between clinical assessments and patients' self-report in depression. *Arch Gen Psychiatry*. 1972;26:546-552.

29 Prusoff BA, Klerman GL, Paykel ES. Pitfalls in the self-report assessment of depression. *Can Psychiatr Assoc J*. 1972;17(Suppl 2):SS101.

30 White J, White K, Razani J. Effects of endogenicity and severity on consistency of standard depression rating scales. *J Clin Psychiatry*. 1984;45:260-261.

31 Sayer NA, Sackheim HA, Moeller JR, et al. The relations between observer rating and self-report of depressive symptomatology. *Psychol Assess*. 1993;5:350-360.

32 Carroll BJ, Fielding JM, Blashki TG. Depression rating scales. A critical review. *Arch Gen Psychiatry*. 1973;28:361-366.

33 Hautzinger M. [The Beck Depression Inventory in clinical practice]. *Nervenarzt*. 1991;62:689-696.

34 Rush AJ, Giles DE, Schlesser MA, et al. The Inventory for Depressive Symptomatology (IDS): preliminary findings. *Psychiatry Res*. 1986;18:65-87.

35 Carroll BJ, Feinberg M, Smouse PE, Rawson SG, Greden JF. The Carroll rating scale for depression. I. Development, reliability and validation. *Br J Psychiatry*. 1981;138:194-200.

36 Rush AJ, Gullion CM, Basco MR, Jarrett RB, Trivedi MH. The Inventory of Depressive Symptomatology (IDS): psychometric properties. *Psychol Med*. 1996;26:477-486.

37 Rush AJ, Trivedi MH, Ibrahim HM, et al. The 16-Item Quick Inventory of Depressive Symptomatology (QIDS), clinician rating (QIDS-C), and self-report (QIDS-SR): a psychometric evaluation in patients with chronic major depression. *Biol Psychiatry*. 2003;54:573-583.

38 Möller HJ, von Zerssen D. Self-rating procedures in the evaluation of antidepressants. *Psychopathology*. 1995;28:291-306.

39 Uher R, Farmer A, Maier W, et al. Measuring depression: comparison and integration of three scales in the GENDEP study. *Psychol Med*. 2008;38:289-300.

40 Möller HJ, Leitner M, Dietzfelbinger T. A linear mathematical model for computerized analyses of mood curves. An empirical investigation on mood courses in depressive and schizophrenic inpatients. *Eur Arch Psychiatry Neurol Sci*. 1987;236:260-268.

41 Morley SJ. Single case methodology in psychopathology therapy. In: Lindsay, SJ. Powell, GW, eds. *Handbook of Clinical Adult Psychology*. London: Routledge; 1994;723-745.

42 Beck AT, Beamesderfer A. Assessment of depression: the depression inventory. In: Pichot P. *Psychological Measurements in Psychopharmacology. Modern Problems in Pharmacopsychiatry*. Vol 7. Basel, Switzerland: Karger; 1974;151-169.

43 Zung WW. The Depression Status Inventory: an adjunct to the Self-Rating Depression Scale. *J Clin Psychol*. 1972;28:539-543.

44 Brown GL, Zung WW. Depression scales: self- or physician-rating? A validation of certain clinically observable phenomena. *Compr Psychiatry*. 1972;13:361-367.

45 Zung WW, Richards CB, Short MJ. Self-rating depression scale in an outpatient clinic. Further validation of the SDS. *Arch Gen Psychiatry*. 1965;13:508-515.

46 Zigmond AS, Snaith RP. The hospital anxiety and depression scale. *Acta Psychiatr Scand*. 1983;67:361-370.

47 Snaith RP, Baugh SJ, Clayden AD, Husain A, Sipple MA. The Clinical Anxiety Scale: an instrument derived from the Hamilton Anxiety Scale. *Br J Psychiatry*. 1982;141:518-523.

48 Wing JK, Cooper JE, Sartorius N. Measurement and classification of psychiatric symptoms; an instruction manual for the PSE and Catego Program. London: Cambridge University Press; 1974.

49 Bjelland I, Dahl AA, Haug TT, Neckelmann D. The validity of the Hospital Anxiety and Depression Scale. An updated literature review. *J Psychosom Res*. 2002;52:69-77.

50 Herrmann C. International experiences with the Hospital Anxiety and Depression Scale--a review of validation data and clinical results. *J Psychosom Res*. 1997;42:17-41.

51 Elliott D. Comparison of three instruments for measuring patient anxiety in a coronary care unit. *Intensive Crit Care Nurs*. 1993;9:195-200.

52 Herrmann C, Scholz KH, Kreuzer H. Psychologisches Screening von einer kardiologischen Akutklinik mit einer deutschen Fassung der "Hospital Anxiety and Depression" (HAD) Skala. *Psychother Psychosom Med Psychol*. 1991;41:83-92.

53 Tignol J. A double-blind, randomized, fluoxetine-controlled, multicenter study of paroxetine in the treatment of depression. *J Clin Psychopharmacol*. 1993;13:18S-22S.

54 Tyrer P, Seivewright N, Murphy S, et al. The Nottingham study of neurotic disorder: comparison of drug and psychological treatments. *Lancet*. 1988;2:235-240.

55 Mykletun A, Stordal E, Dahl AA. Hospital Anxiety and Depression (HAD) scale: factor structure, item analyses and internal consistency in a large population. *Br J Psychiatry*. 2001;179:540-544.

56 Mineka S, Watson D, Clark LA. Comorbidity of anxiety and unipolar mood disorders. *Ann Rev Psychol*. 1998;49:377-412.

57 Herrmann C, Buss U, Snaith RP. HADS-D. Hospital Anxiety and Depression Scale – Deutsche Version. Ein Fragebogen zur Erfassung von Angst und Depressivität in der somatischen Medizin. Testdokumentation und Handanweisung. Bern: Huber; 1995.

58 Derogatis LR, Lipman RS, Covi L. SCL-90: an outpatient psychiatric rating scale--preliminary report. *Psychopharmacol Bull*. 1973;9:13-28.

59 Derogatis LR, Lipman RS, Rickels K, Uhlenhuth EH, Covi L. The Hopkins Symptom Checklist (HSCL): a self-report symptom inventory. *Behav Sci*. 1974;19:1-15.

60 Lipman RS, Covi L, Shapiro AK. The Hopkins Symptom Checklist (HSCL)--factors derived from the HSCL-90. *J Affect Disord.* 1979;1:9-24.

61 Möller HJ, Volz HP, Reimann IW, Stoll KD. Opipramol for the treatment of generalized anxiety disorder: a placebo-controlled trial including an alprazolam-treated group. *J Clin Psychopharmacol.* 2001;21:59-65.

62 Volz HP, Moller HJ, Reimann I, Stoll KD. Opipramol for the treatment of somatoform disorders results from a placebo-controlled trial. *Eur Neuropsychopharmacol.* 2000;10:211-217.

63 Collegium Internationale Psychiatriae Scalarum (CIPS). *Rating scales for Psychiatry.* Weinheim: Beltz; 1990.

64 Cuijpers P, van Straten A, Warmerdam L, Andersson G. Psychotherapy versus the combination of psychotherapy and pharmacotherapy in the treatment of depression: a meta-analysis. *Depress Anxiety.* 2009;26:279-288.

65 Khan A, Khan SR, Shankles EB, Polissar NL. Relative sensitivity of the Montgomery-Asberg Depression Rating Scale, the Hamilton Depression rating scale and the Clinical Global Impressions rating scale in antidepressant clinical trials. *Int Clin Psychopharmacol.* 2002;17:281-285.

66 Naughton MJ, Wiklund I. A critical review of dimension-specific measures of health-related quality of life in cross-cultural research. *Qual Life Res.* 1993;2:397-432.

67 Steer RA, Beck AT, Garrison B. Applications of the Beck Depression Inventory. In: *Assessment of Depression.* N Sartorius, TA Ban, eds. New York: Springer; 1986:123-142.

68 Beck AT, Beck RW. Screening depressed patients in family practice. A rapid technic. *Postgrad Med.* 1972;52:81-85.

69 Kammer D. Eine Untersuchung der psychometrischen Eigenschaften des deutschen Beck-Depressionsinventars (BDI). *Diagnostica.* 1983;29:48-60.

70 Aalto AM, Elovainio M, Kivimaki M, Uutela A, Pirkola S. The Beck Depression Inventory and General Health Questionnaire as measures of depression in the general population: a validation study using the Composite International Diagnostic Interview as the gold standard. *Psychiatry Res.* 2012;197:163-171.

71 Beck AT, Steer RA. Beck Depression Inventory (BDI). In: *Handbook of Psychiatric Measures.* Washington, DC: American Psychiatric Association; 2000.

72 Beck AT, Steer RA, Garbin MG. Psychometric properties of the Beck Depression Inventory. Twenty-five years of evaluation. *Clin Psychol Rev.* 1988;8:77-100.

73 Hautzinger M, Bailer M. *Allgemeine Depressionsskala (ADS).* Göttingen: Beltz Test; 1993.

74 Hautzinger M, Beiler M, Worall H, et al. *Beck-Depressions-Inventar (BDI) Testhandbuch.* 2nd edn. Bern: Huber; 1995.

75 Coles ME, Gibb BE, Heimberg RG. Psychometric evaluation of the Beck Depression Inventory in adults with social anxiety disorder. *Depress Anxiety.* 2001;14:145-148.

76 Steinmeyer EM. [Clinical validity of the Beck Depression Inventory. A facet theoretical re-analysis of multicenter clinical observations]. *Nervenarzt.* 1993;64:717-726.

4. Assessment of pediatric depression

Marta Bravo, María Mayoral, Alejandra Teresa Laorden,
Carmen Moreno

General aspects of pediatric depression scales

Major depressive disorder (MDD) may have a worse prognosis when onset occurs during childhood or adolescence, due to its association with long-term mental and physical health problems that persist into adulthood [1]. In fact, adolescent-onset MDD is associated with more suicide attempts, high risk of recurrence of major depression by young adulthood, early pregnancy, poor school performance, impaired work and social skills, impaired family functioning, and substance abuse during young adulthood [2,3].

Lifetime prevalence of MDD during adolescence is close to 8% and it is more common among girls than boys (11.1% vs 4.3%). Data on point prevalence are more heterogeneous, but the differential distribution prevails, with almost double the prevalence in boys as compared with girls [4]. In young people under the age of 13, the prevalence is significantly lower — approximately 3% between 12 and 14 years of age and much lower in younger children — and equally distributed between the sexes [5]. In medical settings, prevalence figures may even be double [5]. Sub-threshold symptoms may also have a significant impact on the development of social and vocational skills.

Depression in adults is primarily characterized by persistent sad mood or irritability and/ or loss of interest or pleasure in activities that were previously enjoyed [6]. The clinical picture in the juvenile population is quite different and, overall, symptoms of depression vary with age. In children and younger adolescents, somatic symptoms, anxiety, and irritability are more prevalent than sadness, whereas in older adolescents the clinical picture is closer to the adult presentation, with predominance of affective and cognitive symptoms. Furthermore, depressed young people experience high comorbidity rates, including anxiety disorders, substance abuse, disruptive behavior disorders, and medical illnesses [7]. Association with suicidality is particularly prevalent. Some studies have found that 20–24% of adolescents with MDD attempt suicide, whereas 25–66% report suicidal ideation [8,9].

© Springer International Publishing Switzerland 2014

G. Alexopoulos et al., *Guide to Assessment Scales in Major Depressive Disorder*,
DOI 10.1007/978-3-319-04627-3_4

Nevertheless, the majority of depressed young people do not receive any type of treatment and those treated experience delays in the initiation of treatment. This is especially challenging as longer duration of untreated illness in children and adolescents has been linked to more frequent recurrences and greater difficulties with development of social and emotional skills, leading to poor outcomes [10]. Therefore, early detection and intervention may be essential to preventing depression-derived psychosocial and emotional sequelae. In this chapter, several scales that can assist the clinician in screening for depression in children and adolescents, rating its overall severity, and assessing changes in severity over time will be discussed.

Examples of scales in pediatric depression

The Center for Epidemiological Studies Depression Scale for Children
The Center for Epidemiological Studies Depression Scale for Children (CES-DC) is a 20-item (empirically selected) self-report depression questionnaire developed for the screening of depressive symptoms corresponding to different depressive disorders in non-clinical samples [11,12]. It takes an average of 5 minutes to complete and another 5 minutes to rate. The CES-DC uses a multidimensional approach to assess depressive symptoms in children and adolescents 6 to 17 years of age over the past week. It can be used on an individual or group level.

The items consist of simple statements about emotional, cognitive, and behavioral components of depressiveness, drafted in first-person style. Most items are rated on a four-point scale in relation to their incidence during the past week (0 = "not at all"; 1 = "a little"; 2 = "some"; 3 = "a lot"). However, items 4, 8, 12, and 16 are phrased positively, and thus are scored in the opposite order (3 = "not at all"; 2 = "a little"; 1 = "some" ; 0 = "a lot") [12,13]. The total score is the sum of all item scores (ranging from 0 to 60), with higher CES-DC scores indicating increasing levels of depression. A cut-off point of 15 used for the screening of children and adolescents in clinical settings produced a false-positive rate of 41% and a false negative rate of 37% [13]. Studies in non-clinical samples suggest that a higher cutoff is needed [12,13]. The total score is unreliable when more than four items are not answered [14]. Factor analyses have revealed a four-factor structure in the adult version: negative affect, positive affect, somatic, and interpersonal factors [14]. The same factors have been found in adolescents [15].

The CES-DC showed moderate to high correlation with other depression tests such as the Children's Depression Inventory (CDI) (r = 0.44 to r = 0.58) [13,15], but also with depression-like constructs and total scores for emotional and behavioral problems (r = 0.52 for anxiety; r = 0.43 for self-esteem; r = 0.59 for the total score of the Child Behavior Checklist) [14,15], which is a limitation for the discriminant validity of the CES-DC. Internal consistency is generally good, with Cronbach's α ranging from 0.77 to 0.91, [13,16–18], although lower consistency has been reported for younger children than for adolescents and for boys than for girls [12,13]. Test–retest reliability has been analyzed showing r = 0.79 for a 1-week interval in a 15-year-old

Guatemalan population [19], and r = 0.51 for a 2-week interval in child and adolescent patients after discharge [12].

Thus, the CES-DC has moderate-to-good internal reliability and moderate stability in adolescents, with limited utility in children. Its brevity makes it useful as a first-line screening instrument, although due to its low discriminant validity, further assessment is required.

Kutcher Adolescent Depression Scale

The Kutcher Adolescent Depression Scale (KADS) is a short self-report scale for both diagnosing and monitoring the severity of depression in adolescents [20]. There are three forms of the scale: the 6-item, the 11-item, and the 16-item. In its full form, the KADS consists of 16 items covering the core symptoms of adolescent depression, including cognitive, affective, behavioral, psychomotor, and somatic fields. Items are described in standard colloquial language. The scale measures frequency of symptoms over the previous week on a scale from 0 to 3: "hardly ever"; "much of the time"; "most of the time"; and "all of the time." The total score is the sum of all 16 items. There are some exceptions to this coding:

- item 8 (appetite changes) has a dichotomous answer where subjects indicate if their appetite has increased or decreased (this response does not contribute to the total score);
- response options for items 12 (interest in/thoughts re: sex, sexual arousal); and
- item 13 (thoughts/actions regarding suicide/self-harm) are worded slightly differently, but are also listed in ascending order of morbidity, with four response options required in item 12 (from 0 to 3) and five in item 13 (from 0 to 4).

The diagnostic validity of the KADS has been demonstrated in a school-based sample of adolescents [20]. The study used receiver operating characteristic curve analysis to compare the diagnostic validity of the full-length KADS, briefer versions of that scale, and the Beck Depression Inventory (BDI) against the criteria for a major depressive episode from the Mini International Neuropsychiatric Interview. The results showed that a 6-item subscale of the KADS could be used at least as effectively as the BDI to screen for major depressive episodes among school-based adolescents [20].

To investigate which version of the KADS had optimal sensitivity to change, a subsequent study compared the 6-item version, a longer 11-item version, and the full 16-item scale against the clinician-rated Children's Depression Rating Scale-Revised (CDRS-R) [20]. Clinician-rated changes in severity were significantly better corroborated by the 11-item KADS (mean correlation with the CDRS-R, r = 0.69) than by the 6-item KADS (r = 0.62) and at least as well corroborated as by the full-length KADS (r = 0.64) [21]. Furthermore, in terms of mean percentage change in scores from day 0 to day 56, the 11-item KADS (59%) significantly outperformed the full-length KADS (46%) and the CDRS-R (43%) and at least matched the performance of the 6-item KADS (56%) [21]. Thus, the KADS scale ultimately consists of a package with a 6-item version intended for screening and a longer version (either 11 or 16 items) intended for evaluative purposes.

Reynolds Child/Adolescent Depression Scale

The Reynolds Child Depression Scale (RCDS) and the Reynolds Adolescent Depression Scale (RADS) [22,23] are two 30-item self-report questionnaires developed for screening, monitoring, and measuring the severity of depressive symptomatology in children (ages 9–12) and adolescents [18–22], respectively. Both instruments are easy to administer and take no longer than 10 minutes to complete.

Their structures are analogous, using a four-point (1 to 4) response format ("almost never"; "hardly ever"; "sometimes"; and "most of the time"). The tests contain six *critical* items that have been shown to discriminate between depressed and non-depressed individuals. Scores range between 30 and 120 (the higher the score, the more severe the episode). A healthy standardization sample was used to validate mean scores between 52 and 60 [22]. Both a total score of 77 or higher and a score of 3 or 4 on at least four of the six critical items on two consecutive occasions have been proposed as a threshold for significant depression [24].

The RCDS has been found to have excellent internal consistency and reliability [25]. Convergent validity has been reported for the RCDS when correlated with other measures of depression, self-esteem, and anxiety [22]. The RADS has also shown excellent internal reliability and very good stability in young community samples [25,26]. Regarding convergent validity, the RADS shows a correlation of 0.51 with the suicide-ideation question (*"During the last month have you thought about killing yourself?"*), a correlation of 0.55 with the general well-being question (*"In general, how are you feeling?"*), and a correlation of −0.63 with the student happiness question (*"Are you feeling happy or satisfied with your life?"*) [26]. The RADS has also been used to examine the effects and the phenomenology of depression, suicidality, violence, and loss and has served as a model for other depression and suicidality scales.

Despite these advantages, both have some disadvantages derived from their development and predominant use in non-clinical samples, probably related to their weaker ability in monitoring clinical changes and treatment effects. Parent and teacher scores do not agree with child self-ratings. Sensitivity, specificity, and a norm cut-off score in clinical subjects have also not been developed [26].

There is an abbreviated version of the RADS, the RADS-2: Short Form (RADS-2: SF) [27], consisting of ten items used to screen for and measure the severity of depressive symptoms in adolescents 12 to 20 years of age. The RADS-2: SF includes the six critical items from the RADS and four other items selected to reflect mood disorder, loss of interest, and irritability. It takes 2–3 minutes to complete and can be administered in an individual or group setting, making it a useful tool for school guidance counselors and psychologists. The RADS-2: SF has been found to have acceptable reliability and validity and to have psychometric properties comparable to the RADS in a large population of adolescents [28].

Children's Depression Rating Scale–Revised

The CDRS-R is a semi-structured clinician-rated interview developed to assess depression in children 6–12 years of age [29]. It is based on the Hamilton Depression Rating Scale and covers different symptom domains, assessing physical symptoms more deeply than other scales. It includes several items not specific to depression, which limits its discriminant validity. The CDRS-R integrates information from different sources and also takes into account the child's behavior during the interview, which allows for a comprehensive assessment. Although a high degree of clinical expertise is needed for raters, good concordance among examiners has been reported [26]. The clinician is required to produce three different scores: parent and child scores, based on individual interviews with each, and a final summary score. There are 17 symptom areas that are assessed: 14 on a seven-point Likert scale and three on a five-point scale. For the items that use a seven-point scale, a score of 1 or 2 is consistent with subclinical or no symptoms; a score of 3–4 with clinical symptoms; and a score of 5–7 with severe symptoms. For the three items using a five-point scale, a score of 4 or 5 is indicative of severe symptoms. The sum of all 17 items produces the summary score. Scores of ≥40 indicate a high likelihood of a depressive disorder [30].

Normative data were based on a non-clinical sample of children who were interviewed directly, showing good internal consistency (Cronbach's α 0.85), good test-retest reliability (0.89), and good inter-rater reliability (0.92) [29,30]. Although the instrument was designed for use in children, good reliability and validity have been demonstrated in adolescents with depression [31,32]. Internal consistency was good on three consecutive visits (screening: 0.79; baseline: 0.74; exit: 0.92), and total score correlated highly with global severity (0.87–0.93) in a clinical sample of adolescents. Reductions in the CDRS-R total score correlated with improvement scores at exit [31]. In another study conducted with adolescents in primary care settings, scores of ≥30 on the CDRS-R achieved a sensitivity of 83% and a specificity of 84% [32].

The CDRS-R has been widely used in research due to its clinician-rated format, the integration of different sources of information, and its usefulness for monitoring treatment effects. However, rater and time constraints make it less useful in clinical settings.

Featured scale: Children's Depression Inventory

The CDI is one of the most frequently used scales for the screening of depression in children and adolescents [26,33]. It is a self-report instrument covering the core symptoms of depression, based on the BDI, developed for use in children and adolescents between 7 and 17 years of age. Although the CDI was originally created for individual use in clinical settings, it has been expanded to non-clinical settings and the group format. It is written in colloquial language and is easy to understand both for children and adolescents.

The CDI is a norm-referenced test, based on clinical samples [33]. It contains 27 items with three answer options (0: absence of symptoms; 1: mild symptoms; and 2: definite symptoms) covering a temporal framework of two weeks, and a total score ranging from 0 to 54. Following a five-factor solution for children and adolescents, the full-length CDI is divided into five subscales: negative mood, interpersonal problems, ineffectiveness, anhedonia, and negative self-esteem, although a general score is preferred [26]. While a cut-off score of 19 was recommended for authors in non-clinical populations, lower scores have been proposed in clinical samples; recently, a study including children and adolescents found that a cut-off of 16 correctly classified patients with depression, with a sensitivity of 94% and a specificity of 84% [34]. The CDI can also be used as a continuous measure of depressive symptoms, as it has well-established sensitivity to change [35]. Along with the full scale, a short form including 12 items is also available. Parent-rated (17 items) and teacher-rated (12 items) versions have also been developed. Items on both scales are rated from 0 to 3 in order to gather a more comprehensive assessment and are rephrased to emphasize symptoms of depression most likely to be observed.

Regarding psychometric properties, internal consistency evaluated with Cronbach's α ranges from 0.71 to 0.87 [34–36]. Test-retest reliability is highly variable, depending on the time interval between assessments, and is lower in the general population than in clinical samples [37,38]. However, a recent study found good correlation when used 6-months apart (r = 0.73 for children and r= 0.72 for adolescents) [39]. Regarding concurrent validity, the CDI was found to correlate positively with scales measuring anxiety, self-esteem, or hopelessness, and to predict risk of future depression [40]. As for discriminant validity, results were better with semi-structured diagnostic interviews than with clinically-derived diagnosis [41]. Using the CDI with the CDRS-R seems to provide a more accurate diagnostic assessment [28].

A meta-analysis exploring gender and ethnic considerations related to the CDI pointed to an age-by-gender interaction, stressing that boys tend to have higher depression scores at younger ages, while girls' scores are slightly higher in pre-adolescence [42]. Results for ethnic differences were mixed [42]. The CDI is available in 43 languages, although relatively few studies have been performed to validate the translated versions [34]. A Spanish version of the CDI is available for Spanish-speaking populations. The second edition, CDI-2, has been available since 2011 [43].

References

1   Thombs BD, Roseman M, Kloda LA. Depression screening and mental health outcomes in children and adolescents a systematic review protocol. *Syst Rev.* 2012;1:58.

2   Cullen K, Klimes-Dougan B, Kumra S, Schulz SC. Paediatric major depressive disorder: neurobiology and implications for early intervention. *Early Interv Psychiatry.* 2009;3:178-188.

3   Fergusson DM, Woodward LJ. Mental health, educational, and social role outcomes of adolescents with depression. *Arch Gen Psychiatry.* 2002;59:225-231.

4   Cheung AH, Dewa CS: Canadian Community Health Survey: major depressive disorder and suicidality in adolescents. *Health Policy.* 2006;2:76-89.

5   Sharp LK, Lipsky MS. Screening for depression across the lifespan: a review of measures for use in primary care settings. *Am Fam Physician.* 2002;66:1001-1008.

6   *Diagnostic and Statistical Manual of Mental Disorders.* 4th edn. Washington D.C.: American Psychiatric Association; 1994.

7   Moreno C, Arango C, Parellada M, Shaffer D, Bird H. Antidepressants in child and adolescent depression: where are the bugs? *Acta Psychiatr Scand.* 2007;115:184-195.

8   Kovacs M, Goldston D, Gatsonis C. Suicidal behaviors and childhood-onset depressive disorders: a longitudinal investigation. *J Am Acad Child Adolesc Psychiatry.* 1993;32:8-20.

9 Tuisku V, Pelkonen M, Karlsson L, et al.Suicidal ideation, deliberate self-harm behaviour and suicide attempts among adolescent outpatients with depressive mood disorders and comorbid axis I disorders. *Eur Child Adolesc Psychiatr.* 2006;15:199-206.

10 Patton GC, Coffey C, Romaniuk H, et al. The prognosis of common mental disorders in adolescents: a 14-year prospective cohort study. *Lancet.* 2014;S0140-6736.

11 Radloff LS. The CES-D scale: a self-report depression scale research in the general population. *Appl Psychol Meas.* 1977;1:385-401.

12 Weissman MM, Orvaschel H, Padian N. Children's symptom and social functioning self- report scales: comparison of mothers'and children's reports. *J Nerv Ment Dis.* 1980;168:736-740.

13 Faulstich ME, Carey MP, Ruggiero L, Enyart P, Gresham F. Assessment of depression in childhood and adolescence: an evaluation of the Center for Epidemiological Studies Depression Scale for Children (CES-DC). *Am J Psychiatry.* 1986;143:1024-1027.

14 Radloff LS. The CES-D scale: a self-report depression scale for research in the general population. *Appl Psychol Meas.* 1977;1:385-401.

15 Essau CA, Olaya B, Pasha G, Gilvarry C, Bray D. Depressive symptoms among children and adolescents in Iran: a confirmatory factor analytic study of the centre for epidemiological studies depression scale for children. *Child Psychiatry Hum Dev.* 2013;44:123-136.

16 Doerfler LA, Felner RD, Rowlison RT, Raley PA, Evans E. Depression in children and adolescents: a comparative analysis of the utility and construct validity of two assessment measures. *J Consult Clin Psychol.* 1988;56:769-772.

17 Fendrich M, Weissman MM, Warner V. Screening for depressive disorder in children and adolescents: validating the Center for Epidemiologic Studies depression scale for children. *Am J Epidemiol.* 1990;131:538-551.

18 Olsson G, von Knorring AL. Depression among Swedish adoles cents measured by the self-rating scale Center for Epidemiology Studies- depression child (CES-DC). *Eur Child Adolesc Psychiatry.* 1997;6:81-87.

19 Aguilar G, Berganza CE. Confiabilidad test-retest de la Escala de Depresion para Ninos y Adolescentes del Centro de Estudios Epidemiologicos (CES-DC-M) en el diagnostico de la depresión en adolescentes guatemaltecos. *Av Piscol Clin Latinonot.* 1993;11:59-63.

20 LeBlanc JC, Almudevar A, Brooks SJ, Kutcher S. Screening for adolescent depression: comparison of the Kutcher Adolescent Depression Scale with the Beck Depression Inventory. *J Child Adolesc Psychopharmacol.* 2002;12:113-126.

21 Brooks SJ, Krulewicz SP, Kutcher S. The Kutcher Adolescent Depression Scale: assessment of its evaluative properties over the course of an 8-Week pediatric pharmacotherapy trial. *J Child Adolesc Psychopharmacol.* 2003;13:337-349.

22 Reynolds, WM. *Reynolds Child Depression Scale: Professional Manual.* Lutz, FL: Psychological Assessment Resources, Inc;1989.

23 Reynolds WM, Mazza JJ. Reliability and validity of the Reynolds Adolescent Depression Scale with young adolescents. *J Sch Psychol.*1998;36:295-312.

24 Reynolds WM. *RADS Professional Manual.* Odessa, FL: Psychological Assessment Resources; 1986.

25 Walker L, Merry S, Watson PD, Robinson E, Crengle S, Schaaf D. The Reynolds Adolescent Depression Scale in New Zealand adolescents. *Aust NZ J Psychiatry.* 2005;39:136-140.

26 Myers K, Winters NC. Ten-year review of rating scales. II: scales for internalizing disorders. *J Am Acad of Child Adolesc Psychiatry.* 2002;41:634-659.

27 Reynolds WM. *Reynolds Adolescent Depression Scale.* 2nd edn. Short Form. Lutz, Florida: PAR; 2002.

28 Milfont TL, Merry S, Robinson E, Denny S, Crengle S, Ameratunga S. Evaluating the short form of the Reynolds Adolescent Depression Scale in New Zealand adolescents. *Aust NZ J Psychiatry.* 2008;42:950-954.

29 Poznanski EO, Grossman JA, Buchsbaum Y, Banegas M, Freeman L, Gibbons R. Preliminary studies of the reliability and validity of the children's depression rating scale. *J Am Acad Child Psychiatry.* 1984;23:191-197.

30 Poznanski EO, Freeman LN, Mokros HB. Children´s Depression Rating Scale-Revised. *Psychopharmacology Bulletin.* 1985;21:979-989.

31 Mayes TL, Bernstein IH, Haley CL, Kennard, BD, Emslie, GJ. Psychometric Properties of the Children's Depression Rating Scale - Revised in Adolescents. *J Child Adolesc Psychopharmacology*. 2010;20:513-516.

32 Mona M Basker MM, Russell PS, Russell S, Moses PD. Validation of the children's depression rating scale-revised for adolescents in primary-care pediatric use in India. *Indian J Med Sci*. 2010;64:72-80.

33 Kovacs M. The Children's Depression Inventory (CDI). *Psychopharmacol Bull*. 1985;21:995-998.

34 Brooks SJ, Kutcher S. Diagnosis and measurement of adolescent depression: a review of commonly utilized instruments. *J Child Adolesc Psychopharmacol*. 2001;11:341-376.

35 Stone LB, Uhrlass DJ, Gibb BE. Co-rumination and lifetime history of depressive disorders in children. *J Clin Child Adolesc Psychol*. 2010;39:597-602.

36 Kovacs M, Feinberg TL, Crouse-Novak MA, Paulauskas SL, Finkelstein R. Depressive disorders in childhood. I. A longitudinal prospective study of characteristics and recovery. *Arch Gen Psychiatry*. 1984;41:229-237.

37 Kazdin AE. Children's Depression Scale: validation with child psychiatric inpatients. *J Child Psychol Psychiatry*. 1987;28:29-41

38 Sorensen MJ, Frydenberg M, Thastum M, Thomsen PH. The Children's Depression Inventory and classification of major depressive disorder: validity and reliability of the Danish version. *Eur Child Adolesc Psychiatry*. 1984;14:328-334.

39 Cole DA, Martin NC. The longitudinal structure of the Children's Depression Inventory: testing a latent trait-state model. *Psychol Assess*. 2005;17:144-155.

40 Canals J, Domènech-Llaberia E, Fernández-Ballart J, Martí-Henneberg C. Predictors of depression at eighteen. A 7-year follow-up study in a Spanish nonclinical population. *Eur Child Adolesc Psychiatry*. 2002;5:20-28.

41 Timbremont B, Braet C, Dreesen L. Assessing depression in youth: relation between the Children's Depression Inventory and a structured interview. *J Clin Child Adolesc Psychol*. 2004;33:149-157.

42 Twenge JM, Nolen-Hoeksema S. Age, gender, race, socioeconomic status, and birth cohort differences on the children's depression inventory: a meta-analysis. *J Abnorm Psychol*. 2002;111:578-588.

43 Kovacs M. Spanish Children's Depression Inventory (CDI) 2. North Tonawanda, NY: Multihealth Systems, Inc; 2011.

5. Assessment scales for geriatric patients

George S. Alexopoulos

General aspects of depression scales for geriatric patients

Late-life depression causes suffering, family disruption, and disability, worsens the outcomes of many medical illnesses, and increases mortality [1]. Depression preferentially afflicts older adults with cognitive impairment and high medical burden [2]. Part of the reason is that vulnerability to late-life depression is principally caused by aging-related and disease-related processes, including arteriosclerosis, inflammatory, endocrine, and immune changes that compromise the integrity of frontolimbic pathways [1]. Heredity is an additional vulnerability factor. Chronic stress resulting from financial difficulties, disability, isolation, relocation, caregiving, and bereavement, causes physiological changes, which further increase vulnerability to depression or trigger depression in already vulnerable older adults.

Symptom assessment

Cognitive impairment is ubiquitous in late-life depression. Approximately 20% of older adults with dementia also have major depression, and an additional 15% have milder depressive syndromes. Depression is often a prodrome and a risk factor for dementia [3,4]. Even older patients with major depression, but without dementia, often experience disturbances in attention, speed of mental processing, and executive function [5]. These deficits improve after remission of late-life major depression but still remain abnormal [6,7]. In some older patients with depression, cognitive dysfunction can be severe enough to meet the criteria for dementia, but subsides when the symptoms and signs of depression remit. This 'reversible' dementia syndrome is usually mild and occurs in the context of severe late-onset depression [8]. More than 40% of depressed older patients with reversible dementia develop an irreversible dementia syndrome during follow-up, suggesting that the pathophysiological changes of depression unmask a subclinical dementia process (ie, depression uncovered the patients' decreased reserve cognitive capacity) [8]. Patients with depression who do not go on

© Springer International Publishing Switzerland 2014   43
G. Alexopoulos et al., *Guide to Assessment Scales in Major Depressive Disorder*,
DOI 10.1007/978-3-319-04627-3_5

to develop dementia may have a non-progressive brain lesion compromising circuitry related to mood and cognitive symptoms. Another possibility is that their cognitive dysfunction is an integral part of severe geriatric depression because cognitive dysfunction can be a primary sign of depression rather than an indirect behavioral consequence of the affective symptoms of depression. The frequent presence of depression in patients with reversible or irreversible dementia underscores the need for a reliable assessment method of depression in this population.

Various factors complicate the assessment of depression in patients with cognitive impairment or dementia. Some symptoms of depression overlap with behavioral manifestations of dementia, including apathy and loss of initiative. In patients with dementia, depressive symptoms may fluctuate over time or fail to meet criteria for intensity, duration, or functional impact required for a diagnosis of major depression. The clinical presentation of depressive symptoms and signs may change with the progression of Alzheimer's disease [9].

Another problem in ascertaining depressive symptoms is the difficulty of cognitively impaired and patients with dementia to accurately report depressive symptoms. In fact, the identification of depressive symptomatology in patients with dementia varies markedly depending on whether it is based on reports from patients, caregivers, or trained observers [10–12]. Sampling from psychiatric settings is likely to result in higher rates of depression than in population-based samples of patients with dementia. As a result, the prevalence of depressive disorders in patients with dementia ranges from 0–87% [13]. Patient inability to communicate coherently may increase reliance on behavior alone in assessing depression. Combining a patient interview with information obtained by caregivers and using depression scales that focus on symptoms not shared by the depression and the dementia syndromes is helpful in assessing depressive symptoms and signs of older adults with varying degrees of cognitive dysfunction [10].

Examples of observer rating scales for geriatric patients

Self-rated scales
The Beck Depression Inventory (BDI) and the Zung Self-Rating Depression Scale have been used in cognitively unimpaired subjects and those with mild dementia [14–17]. The BDI correlated well with scores on the Hamilton Depression Rating Scale (HAM-D) in both unaffected patients and patients with mild dementia [16]. However, 23% of subjects with mild dementia may be unable to complete the Zung Self-Rating Depression Scale [17].

The Geriatric Depression Scale (GDS) was developed with the goal to discriminate depressive symptoms from complaints often reported by non-depressed older adults [18]. The GDS does not assess vegetative symptoms of depression because some such symptoms often occur in normal elders. The GDS consists of 30 questions. An abbreviated 15-item scale also exists. The "yes/no" question format makes the GDS accessible to the elderly population. Although the GDS was originally designed as a self-administered test, it can also be used in a rater-administered format and by telephone [19].

The GDS was initially validated in depression and among normal older adults living in the community [18]. A cut-off score of 11 on the GDS identifies late-life depression with a sensitivity of 84% and a 95% specificity rate, while a cut-off score of 14 has a sensitivity of 80% and a specificity of 100% [18]. The GDS has been validated in diverse older populations. It has an acceptable performance in older medical patients [20,21]. The GDS is an accurate screening test for depression in cognitively intact elderly outpatients, but may not perform well in populations that include large numbers of cognitively impaired patients [22,23]. Approximately 50% of nursing home residents are unable to rate the GDS mainly because of cognitive impairment [24,25]. In institutionalized patients, a GDS cut-off score of 13 was only 47% sensitive and 75% specific in screening for depression [26]. Another study of nursing home residents showed that a GDS cut-off score of 10 or greater identified depression with a sensitivity of 63% and a specificity of 83% [27]. When those with a mini-mental state examination (MMSE) score greater or equal to 15 were included, the sensitivity and specificity of GDS improved to 84% and 91%, respectively. Worse memory was associated with more self-reported depressive symptoms [28]. Alzheimer patients who disavow cognitive deficits also tend to disavow depressive symptoms. These observations suggest that the performance of GDS may be influenced both by memory impairment and by patients' inability to identify their cognitive impairment. In sum, the GDS-30 is a reliable screening tool for depressive symptoms in patients without dementia and with mild cognitive impairment, but not in patients with moderate or severe dementia [29–31].

Interviewer-rated scales

Scales such as the HAM-D and the Montgomery-Åsberg Depression Rating Scale (MADRS) are broadly used to quantify severity of depression. Potential limitations of the HAM-D are its scoring system that mixes frequency and severity of symptoms, its heterogeneous factor structure, and its emphasis on somatic symptoms that are common even in non-depressed older adults. The HAM-D utilizes information from a patient interview and requires sufficient comprehension and judgment to answer questions related to affect and ideation. Further, valid information about sleep, eating, and other physiological functions can be obtained only from patients with intact memory. Thus, patients with moderate or severe dementia cannot be reliably evaluated on the basis of information derived solely from a HAM-D structured interview. The HAM-D has been inadequately validated in older adults [32].

The MADRS consists of ten items, each rated across six grades. The MADRS does not include somatic items likely to be endorsed by non-depressed older adults. The MADRS has been validated in younger populations and its performance compared against other rating scales [33]. However, its non-somatic items require accurate understanding and rather complex judgments that may be difficult to be made by patients with dementia. Nonetheless, there is evidence that the MADRS may correctly identify depression in outpatients of a memory clinic and in patients with dementia when administered to patients' caregivers [34–36].

The Alzheimer's Disease Assessment Scale

The Alzheimer's Disease Assessment Scale (ADAS) was specifically designed for the assessment of patients with Alzheimer's disease [37]. It consists of a cognitive component and a non-cognitive component. The non-cognitive behavioral component of ADAS consists of clinician ratings of:

- depression;
- tearfulness;
- restlessness;
- appetite;
- hallucinations;
- delusions;
- pacing;
- concentration; and
- tremor.

It is scored on the basis of patient observation and an interview of an informant. While it circumvents most of the difficulties associated with interview scales, the behavior component of ADAS includes only a small number of depressive signs and symptoms and may, therefore, be insensitive in detecting mild depression. Moreover, the ADAS was developed primarily for assessment of patients with moderate or severe dementia whose cognitive impairments were expected to be progressive ; thus, it may be less useful in evaluating depressive symptoms in patients with mild dementia or in patients whose cognitive functioning improves.

Depression Signs Scale

This rating scale consists of nine items whose ratings are based exclusively on patient observation [38]. The Depression Signs Scale (DSS) has satisfactory inter-rater reliability, but its internal consistency and validity require further testing. The DSS can be useful for rating depression in subjects with severe dementia. However, this instrument may be less suitable for assessing depression in patients with mild or moderate dementia, as it covers a relatively narrow range of depressive manifestations and does not include items that require interaction with the subject. Therefore, the DSS may fail to assess important aspects of the depressive syndrome in patients with mild depression.

Neuropsychiatric Inventory

The Neuropsychiatric Inventory (NPI) was developed to assess ten behavioral domains often disturbed in patients with dementia [39], such as:

- delusions;
- hallucinations;

- dysphoria;
- anxiety;
- agitation/aggression;
- euphoria;
- disinhibition;
- rritability/lability;
- apathy; and
- aberrant motor behavior.

The NPI is a rater-administrated instrument based on structured interview of the patient's caregiver. The assessment of each domain starts with a gateway question. If the response to the gateway question is affirmative, the rater asks seven to nine follow-up questions on specific symptoms (part of this domain). Any endorsed symptom is rated on a four-point frequency scale as well as a three-point severity scale. The total subscale score is the product of frequency and severity scores.

A major asset of the NPI is its brevity. However, the cost of brevity is a less complete assessment of the depressive syndrome. Further, some depressive symptoms may be missed, especially when the gateway questions are answered negatively. To overcome these limitations the Neuropsychiatric Inventory-Clinician Rating Scale (NPI-C) has been developed, which expands the NPI domains and items and relies on a clinician-rating methodology [40]. The convergent validity of the NPI-C was tested against the Cornell Scale for Depression in Dementia (CSDD) and found to be satisfactory (r=0.61).

Dementia Mood Assessment Scale

The Dementia Mood Assessment Scale (DMAS) is a 24-item scale that assesses observable mood functional capacities of patients with dementia [41]. Some of the DMAS items are derived from HAM-D but its items were formulated in a way that they can be assessed objectively. The first 17 items are the most representative of mood symptoms and signs in dementia. The remaining seven items are related to the severity of dementia but are not intended to assess mood per se. The initial validation of DMAS was based on a semi-structured patient interview and patient observation through a one-way mirror. The 17-item dementia mood scale was not influenced by global functional or cognitive impairment, suggesting that this subscale does not simply reflect severity of dementia. In contrast, the last seven items of the DMAS were correlated with global impairment scores.

Featured scale: Cornell Scale for Depression in Dementia

The CSDD is a 19-item instrument specifically designed for the rating of symptoms and signs of depression in patients with dementia [10,42] (Appendix D). The items were selected after reviewing the literature on the phenomenology of depression in patients with [37,43] and without [44] dementia, and obtaining information from a questionnaire answered by 11 geriatric psychiatrists from the Cornell University Medical College and other experts in the field. Items were constructed so that they could be rated primarily on the basis of observation. Phobias, obsessions, and complex depressive ideation were not included in the scale because they usually require reliable self-reporting. To simplify the use of the scale, the severity of each item is rated according to three explicitly defined grades (ie, absent, mild/intermittent, and severe).

How to use the Cornell Scale for Depression in Dementia

The CSDD is administered in two steps: the clinician interviews the patient's caregiver on each of the 19 items of the CSDD and then briefly interviews the patient. The interview is guided by a detailed Administration Manual that describes each item and guides the interviewer (Appendix D). The clinician is free to use additional descriptions to help the caregiver understand the meaning of each item. The caregiver is instructed to base his/her report on observations of the patient's behavior during the week prior to interview.

Two of the items, "loss of interest" and "lack of energy," require not only that the patient is less involved in usual activities or has less energy during the week prior to interview, but also that changes in these behaviors occurred relatively acutely (ie, over a period of less than 1 month). In these two items, the caregiver is initially asked to describe the patient's behavior during the week prior to interview and, then, is asked to provide information about the onset of behavioral changes that may have occurred earlier. The item on weight loss is based entirely on information about the patient's weight during the month preceding the interview.

During the interview with the caregiver, the clinician assigns preliminary scores to each item of the CSDD. Next, the clinician briefly interviews the patient using CSDD items as a basis for inquiry and observation, but does not necessarily confine himself/herself to these questions. If there is a large discrepancy between the clinician's observations and the caregiver's report on any item, the clinician interviews the caregiver and/or the patient again and attempts to clarify the reason for disagreement. After this process, the CSDD is scored on the basis of the clinician's final judgment.

Quality and characteristics of the Cornell Scale for Depression in Dementia

The CSDD was initially validated in elderly patients (with and without dementia) [10,42]. In more recent studies, the CSDD performed well in distinguishing depressed from non-depressed long-term care patients [35]. The CSDD consistently identified depression in outpatients with Alzheimer's dementia and found to be a valid screening tool for depression in older adults with and without dementia [30,34]. CSDD scores at baseline was a risk factor for later development of depression in long-term care facilities [45]. The CSDD has been found sensitive to change with treatment [46]. In outpatients with probable Alzheimer's disease, principal-factors analysis of the CSDD identified four factors [47]:

- general depression (lack of reactivity to pleasant events, poor self-esteem, pessimism, loss of interest, physical complaints, psychomotor retardation, sadness);

- rhythm disturbances (difficulty falling asleep, multiple night awakenings, early morning awakenings, weight loss, diurnal variation of mood);
- agitation/psychosis (agitation, mood-congruent delusions, suicide); and
- negative symptoms (appetite loss, weight loss, lack of energy, loss of interest, lack of reactivity to pleasant events).

Receiver-operated characteristics analyses showed that a cut-off score greater than 7 might be optimal in distinguishing depressed from non-depressed patients with dementia [48]. More than 30% of long-term care patients had a CSDD score >7 [49]. However, the cut-off score associated with depression may be influenced by cultural factors; for example, a higher cut-off score distinguished depressed from non-depressed older patients more often in Brazilian than in Norwegian samples [50,51].

References

1 Alexopoulos GS. Depression in the elderly. *Lancet*. 2005;365:1961-1970.

2 Blazer DG. Depression in late-life: review and commentary. *J Gerontol A Biol Sci Med Sci*. 2003;58:249-265.

3 Yaffe K, Blackwell T, Gore R, et al. Depressive symptoms and cognitive decline in nondemented elderly women: a prospective study. *Arch Gen Psychiatry*. 1999;56:425-430.

4 Gao Y, Huang C, Zhao K, et al. Depression as a risk factor for dementia and mild cognitive impairment: a meta-analysis of longitudinal studies. *Int J Geriatr Psychiatry*. 2013;28:441-449.

5 Lockwood KA, Alexopoulos GS, van Gorp WG. Executive dysfunction in geriatric depression. *Am J Psychiatry*. 2002;159:1119-1126.

6 Murphy CF, Alexopoulos GS. Longitudinal association of initiation/perseveration and severity of geriatric depression. *Am J Geriatr Psychiatry*. 2004;12:50-56.

7 Nebes RD, Pollock BG, Houck PR, et al. Persistence of cognitive impairment in geriatric patients following antidepressant treatment: a randomized, double-blind clinical trial with nortriptyline and paroxetine. *J Psychiatr Res*. 2003;37:99-108.

8 Alexopoulos GS, Meyers BS, Young RC, Mattis S, Kakuma T. The course of geriatric depression with "reversible dementia": a controlled study. *Am J Psychiatry*. 1993;150:1693-1699.

9 Forsell Y, Jorm AF, Winblad B. Variation in psychiatric and behavioural symptoms at different stages of dementia: data from physicians' examinations and informants' reports. *Dementia*. 1993;4:282-286.

10 Alexopoulos GS, Abrams RC, Young RC, Shamoian CA. Cornell Scale for Depression in Dementia. *Biol Psychiatry*. 1988;23:271-284.

11 Burke WJ, Roccaforte WH, Wengel SP, et al. Disagreement in the reporting of depressive symptoms between patients with dementia of the Alzheimer type and their collateral sources. *Am J Geriatr Psychiatry*. 1998;6:308-319.

12 Wongpakaran N, Wongpakaran T, van Reekum R. Discrepancies in Cornell Scale for Depression in Dementia (CSDD) items between residents and caregivers, and the CSDD's factor structure. *Clin Interv Aging*. 2013;8:641-648.

13 Alexopoulos GS, Abrams RC. Depression in Alzheimer's disease. *Psychiatr Clin North Am*. 1991;14:327-340.

14 Beck AT, Ward CH, Mendelson M, Mock J, Erbaugh J. An inventory for measuring depression. *Arch Gen Psychiatry*. 1961;4:561-571.

15 Zung WW. A Self-Rating Depression Scale. *Arch Gen Psychiatry*. 1965;12:63-70.

16 Miller NE. The measurement of mood in senile brain disease: examiner ratings and self-reports. In: Cole JO, Barrett JE, eds. *Psychopathology of the Aged*. New York: Raven Press; 1980.

17 Knesevich JW, Martin RL, Berg L, Danziger W. Preliminary report on affective symptoms in the early stages of senile dementia of the Alzheimer type. *Am J Psychiatry.* 1983;140:233-235.

18 Yesavage JA, Brink TL, Rose TL, et al. Development and validation of a geriatric depression screening scale: a preliminary report. *J Psychiatr Res.* 1982;17:37-49.

19 Burke WJ, Roccaforte WH, Wengel SP, Conley DM, Potter JF. The reliability and validity of the Geriatric Depression Rating Scale administered by telephone. *J Am Geriatr Soc.* 1995;43:674-679.

20 Rapp SR, Parisi SA, Walsh DA, Wallace CE. Detecting depression in elderly medical inpatients. *J Consult Clin Psychol.* 1988;56:509-513.

21 Koenig HG, Meador KG, Cohen HJ, Blazer DG. Self-rated depression scales and screening for major depression in the older hospitalized patient with medical illness. *J Am Geriatr Soc.* 1988;36:699-706.

22 Burke WJ, Houston MJ, Boust SJ, Roccaforte WH. Use of the Geriatric Depression Scale in dementia of the Alzheimer type. *J Am Geriatr Soc.* 1989;37:856-860.

23 Burke WJ, Nitcher RL, Roccaforte WH, Wengel SP. A prospective evaluation of the Geriatric Depression Scale in an outpatient geriatric assessment center. *J Am Geriatr Soc.* 1992;40:1227-1230.

24 Lesher EL, Whelihan WM. Reliability of mental status instruments administered to nursing home residents. *J Consult Clin Psychol.* 1986;54:726-727.

25 Parmelee PA, Katz IR, Lawton MP. Depression among institutionalized aged: assessment and prevalence estimation. *J Gerontol.* 1989;44:M22-M29.

26 Kafonek S, Ettinger WH, Roca R, et al. Instruments for screening for depression and dementia in a long-term care facility. *J Am Geriatr Soc.* 1989;37:29-34.

27 McGivney SA, Mulvihill M, Taylor B. Validating the GDS depression screen in the nursing home. *J Am Geriatr Soc.* 1994;42:490-492.

28 Feher EP, Larrabee GJ, Crook TH, 3rd. Factors attenuating the validity of the Geriatric Depression Scale in a dementia population. *J Am Geriatr Soc.* 1992;40:906-909.

29 Debruyne H, Van Buggenhout M, Le Bastard N, et al. Is the geriatric depression scale a reliable screening tool for depressive symptoms in elderly patients with cognitive impairment? *Int J Geriatr Psychiatry.* 2009;24:556-562.

30 Korner A, Lauritzen L, Abelskov K, et al. The Geriatric Depression Scale and the Cornell Scale for Depression in Dementia. A validity study. *Nord J Psychiatry.* 2006;60:360-364.

31 Bonin-Guillaume S, Clement JP, Chassain AP, Leger JM. [Psychometric evaluation of depression in the elderly subject: which instruments? What are the future perspectives?]. *Encephale.* 1995;21:25-34.

32 Lichtenberg PA, Marcopulos BA, Steiner DA, Tabscott JA. Comparison of the Hamilton Depression Rating Scale and the Geriatric Depression Scale: detection of depression in dementia patients. *Psychol Rep.* 1992;70:515-521.

33 Maier W, Heuser I, Philipp M, Frommberger U, Demuth W. Improving depression severity assessment--II. Content, concurrent and external validity of three observer depression scales. *J Psychiatr Res.* 1988;22:13-19.

34 Muller-Thomsen T, Arlt S, Mann U, Mass R, Ganzer S. Detecting depression in Alzheimer's disease: evaluation of four different scales. *Arch Clin Neuropsychol.* 2005;20:271-276.

35 Leontjevas R, van Hooren S, Mulders A. The Montgomery-Asberg Depression Rating Scale and the Cornell Scale for Depression in Dementia: a validation study with patients exhibiting early-onset dementia. *Am J Geriatr Psychiatry.* 2009;17:56-64.

36 Leontjevas R, Gerritsen DL, Vernooij-Dassen MJ, Smalbrugge M, Koopmans RT. Comparative validation of proxy-based Montgomery-Asberg depression rating scale and cornell scale for depression in dementia in nursing home residents with dementia. *Am J Geriatr Psychiatry.* 2012;20:985-993.

37 Mohs RC, Rosen WG, Davis KL. The Alzheimer's disease assessment scale: an instrument for assessing treatment efficacy. *Psychopharmacol Bull.* 1983;19:448-450.

38 Katona CL, Aldridge CR. The dexamethasone suppression test and depressive signs in dementia. *J Affect Disord.* 1985;8:83-89.

39 Cummings JL, Mega M, Gray K, Rosenberg-Thompson S, Carusi DA, Gornbein J. The Neuropsychiatric Inventory: comprehensive assessment of psychopathology in dementia. *Neurology.* 1994;44:2308-2314.

40 de Medeiros K, Robert P, Gauthier S, et al. The Neuropsychiatric Inventory-Clinician rating scale (NPI-C): reliability and validity of a revised assessment of neuropsychiatric symptoms in dementia. *Int Psychogeriatr.* 2010;22:984-994.

41 Sunderland T, Alterman IS, Yount D, et al. A new scale for the assessment of depressed mood in demented patients. *Am J Psychiatry.* 1988;145:955-959.

42 Alexopoulos GS, Abrams RC, Young RC, Shamoian CA. Use of the Cornell scale in nondemented patients. *J Am Geriatr Soc.* 1988;36:230-236.

43 Roth M. The natural history of mental disorder in old age. *J Ment Sci.* 1955;101:281-301.

44 Nelson JC, Charney DS. The symptoms of major depressive illness. *Am J Psychiatry.* 1981;138:1-13.

45 McCusker J, Cole MG, Voyer P, et al. Observer rated depression in long-term care: Frequency and risk factors. *Arch Gerontol Geriatr.* 2013;pii: S0167-4943.

46 Cummings J, Mega M, Gray K, et al. Neuropsychiatric Inventory. In: Rush AJ, ed. *Handbook of Psychiatric Measures.* Washington, DC: American Psychiatric Association; 2000:405-407.

47 Harwood DG, Ownby RL, Barker WW, Duara R. The factor structure of the Cornell Scale for Depression in Dementia among probable Alzheimer's disease patients. *Am J Geriatr Psychiatry.* 1998;6:212-220.

48 Vida S, Des Rosiers P, Carrier L, Gauthier S. Depression in Alzheimer's disease: receiver operating characteristic analysis of the Cornell Scale for Depression in Dementia and the Hamilton Depression Scale. *J Geriatr Psychiatry Neurol.* 1994;7:159-162.

49 Iden KR, Engedal K, Hjorleifsson S, Ruths S. Prevalence of depression among recently admitted long-term care patients in Norwegian nursing homes: associations with diagnostic workup and use of antidepressants. *Dement Geriatr Cogn Disord.* 2013;37:154-162.

50 Knapskog AB, Portugal Mda G, Barca ML, et al. A cross-cultural comparison of the phenotype of depression as measured by the Cornell Scale and the MADRS in two elderly outpatient populations. *J Affect Disord.* 2013;144:34-41.

51 Portugal Mda G, Coutinho ES, Almeida C, et al. Validation of Montgomery-Asberg Rating Scale and Cornell Scale for Depression in Dementia in Brazilian elderly patients. *Int Psychogeriatr.* 2012;24:1291-1298.

Appendix A

Hamilton Depression Rating Scale, 21-item version

Hamilton Depression Rating Scale (HAM-D), 21-item version

1. Depressed Mood (sadness, hopeless, helpless, worthless)	
Absent	0
These feeling states indicated only on questioning	1
These feeling states spontaneously reported verbally	2
Communicates feeling states non-verbally – ie, through facial expression, posture, voice, and tendency to weep	3
Patient reports *VIRTUALLY ONLY* these feeling states in his spontaneous verbal and non-verbal communication	4
2. Feelings of Guilt	
Absent	0
Self-reproach, feels he has let people down	1
Ideas of guilt or rumination over past errors or sinful deeds	2
Present illness is a punishment. Delusions of guilt	3
Hears accusatory or denunciatory voices and/or experiences threatening visual hallucinations	4
3. Suicide	
Absent	0
Feels life is not worth living	1
Wishes he were dead or any thoughts of possible death to self	2
Suicidal ideas or gesture	3
Attempts at suicide (any serious attempt rates 4)	4

Hamilton Depression Rating Scale (HAM-D), 21-item version (continued overleaf)

© Springer International Publishing Switzerland 2014
G. Alexopoulos et al., *Guide to Assessment Scales in Major Depressive Disorder*,
DOI 10.1007/978-3-319-04627-3

Hamilton Depression Rating Scale (HAM-D), 21-item version (continued)

4. Insomnia Early	
No difficulty falling asleep	0
Complains of occasional difficulty falling asleep – ie, more than 1/2 hour	1
Complains of nightly difficulty falling asleep	2
5. Insomnia Middle	
No difficulty	0
Patient complains of being restless and disturbed during the night	1
Waking during the night – any getting out of bed rates 2 (except for purposes of voiding)	2
6. Insomnia Late	
No difficulty	0
Waking in early hours of the morning but goes back to sleep	1
Unable to fall asleep again if he gets out of bed	2
7. Work and Activities	
No difficulty	0
Thoughts and feelings of incapacity, fatigue or weakness related to activities, work or hobbies	1
Loss of interest in activity, hobbies or work – either directly reported by patient, or indirect in listlessness, indecision and vacillation (feels he has to push self to work or activities)	2
Decrease in actual time spent in activities or decrease in productivity	3
Stopped working because of present illness	4
8. Retardation: Psychomotor **(slowness of thought and speech; impaired ability to concentrate; decreased motor activity)**	
Normal speech and thought	0
Slight retardation at interview	1
Obvious retardation at interview	2
Interview difficult	3
Complete stupor	4
9. Agitation	
None	0
Fidgetiness	1
Playing with hands, hair, etc	2
Moving about, can't sit still	3
Hand wringing, nail biting, hair-pulling, biting of lips	4

Hamilton Depression Rating Scale (HAM-D), 21-item version (continued opposite)

Hamilton Depression Rating Scale (HAM-D), 21-item version (continued)

10. Anxiety (psychological)	
No difficulty	0
Subjective tension and irritability	1
Worrying about minor matters	2
Apprehensive attitude apparent in face or speech	3
Fears expressed without questioning	4

11. Anxiety Somatic: Physiological concomitants of anxiety (effects of autonomic overactivity, "butterflies," indigestion, stomach cramps, belching, diarrhea, palpitations, hyperventilation, paresthesia, sweating, flushing, tremor, headache, urinary frequency). Avoid asking about possible medication side effects (ie, dry mouth, constipation)

Absent	0
Mild	1
Moderate	2
Severe	3
Incapacitating	4

12. Somatic Symptoms (gastrointestinal)	
None	0
Loss of appetite but eating without encouragement from others. Food intake about normal	1
Difficulty eating without urging from others. Marked reduction of appetite and food intake	2

13. Somatic Symptoms General	
None	0
Heaviness in limbs, back or head. Backache, headache, or muscle aches. Loss of energy and fatigability	1
Any clear-cut symptom rates "2"	2

14. Genital Symptoms (symptoms such as loss of libido; impaired sexual performance; menstrual disturbances)

Absent	0
Mild	1
Severe	2

15. Hypochondriasis	
Not present	0
Self-absorption (bodily)	1
Preoccupation with health	2
Frequent complaints, requests for help	3
Hypochondriacal delusions	4

Hamilton Depression Rating Scale (HAM-D), 21-item version (continued overleaf)

Hamilton Depression Rating Scale (HAM-D), 21-item version (continued)

16. Loss of weight	
No weight loss	0
Probable weight loss associated with present illness	1
Definite (according to patient) weight loss	2
Not assessed	3
17. Insight	
Acknowledges being depressed and ill	0
Acknowledges illness but attributes cause to bad food, climate, overwork, virus, need for rest	1
Denies being ill at all	3
18. Diurnal variation	
Note whether symptoms are worse in morning or evening. If no diurnal variation, mark 0	
No variation	0
Worse in AM	1
Worse in PM	2
When present, mark the severity of the variation. Mark "None" if no variation	
None	0
Mild	1
Severe	2
19. Depersonalization and derealisation (eg, feelings of unreality, nihilistic ideas)	
Absent	0
Mild	1
Moderate	2
Severe	3
Incapacitating	4
20. Paranoid symptoms	
None	0
Suspicious	1
Ideas of reference	2
Delusions of reference and persecution	3
21. Obsessional and compulsive symptoms	
Absent	0
Mild	1
Severe	2

Hamilton Depression Rating Scale (HAM-D), 21-item version. Reproduced with permission from Hamilton M. A rating scale for depression. *J Neurol Neurosurg Psychiatry.* 1960;23:56-62 ©BMJ.

Appendix B

Montgomery-Åsberg Depression Rating Scale

The rating should be based on a clinical interview moving from broadly phrased questions about symptoms to more detailed ones which allow a precise rating of severity. The rater must decide whether the rating lies on the defined scale steps (0, 2, 4, 6) or between them (1, 3, 5).

It is important to remember that it is only on rare occasions that a depressed patient is encountered who cannot be rated on the items in the scale. If definite answers cannot be elicited from the patient, all relevant clues and information from other sources should be used as a basis for the rating, in line with customary clinical practice.

Montgomery-Åsberg Depression Rating Scale

1. Apparent Sadness	
	Representing despondency, gloom and despair (more than just ordinary transient low spirits) reflected in speech, facial expression, and posture. Rate by depth and inability to brighten up
0	No sadness
1	
2	Looks dispirited but does brighten up without difficulty
3	
4	Appears sad and unhappy most of the time
5	
6	Looks miserable all the time. Extremely despondent
2. Reported Sadness	
	Representing reports of depressed mood, regardless of whether it is reflected in appearance or not. Includes low spirits, despondency or the feeling of being beyond help and without hope
0	Occasional sadness in keeping with the circumstances
1	

Montgomery-Åsberg Depression Rating Scale (continued overleaf)

© Springer International Publishing Switzerland 2014
G. Alexopoulos et al., *Guide to Assessment Scales in Major Depressive Disorder*,
DOI 10.1007/978-3-319-04627-3

Montgomery-Åsberg Depression Rating Scale (continued)

2	Sad or low but brightens up without difficulty
3	
4	Pervasive feelings of sadness or gloominess. The mood is still influenced by external circumstances
5	
6	Continuous or unvarying sadness, misery or despondency

3. Inner Tension

	Representing feelings of ill-defined discomfort, edginess, inner turmoil, mental tension mounting to either panic, dread or anguish. Rate according to intensity, frequency, duration and the extent of reassurance called for
0	Placid. Only fleeting inner tension
1	
2	Occasional feelings of edginess and ill-defined discomfort
3	
4	Continuous feelings of inner tension or intermittent panic which the patient can only master with some difficulty
5	
6	Unrelenting dread or anguish. Overwhelming panic

4. Reduced Sleep

	Representing the experience of reduced duration or depth of sleep compared to the subject's own normal pattern when well
0	Sleeps as normal.
1	
2	Slight difficulty dropping off to sleep or slightly reduced, light, or fitful sleep
3	
4	Moderate stiffness and resistance
5	
6	Sleep reduced or broken by at least 2 hours

5. Reduced Appetite

	Representing the feeling of a loss of appetite compared with when well. Rate by loss of desire for food or the need to force oneself to eat
0	Normal or increased appetite
1	
2	Slightly reduced appetite
3	

Montgomery-Åsberg Depression Rating Scale (continued opposite)

Montgomery-Åsberg Depression Rating Scale (continued)

4	No appetite. Food is tasteless
5	
6	Needs persuasion to eat at all

6. Concentration Difficulties

	Representing difficulties in collecting one's thoughts mounting to an incapacitating lack of concentration
0	No difficulties in concentrating
1	
2	Occasional difficulties in collecting one's thoughts
3	
4	Difficulties in concentrating and sustaining thought which reduced ability to read or hold a conversation
5	
6	Unable to read or converse without great difficulty

7. Lassitude

	Representing difficulty in getting started or slowness in initiating and performing everyday activities
0	Hardly any difficulty in getting started. No sluggishness
1	
2	Difficulties in starting activities
3	
4	Difficulties in starting simple routine activities which are carried out with effort
5	
6	Complete lassitude. Unable to do anything without help

8. Inability to Feel

	Representing the subjective experience of reduced interest in the surroundings or activities that normally give pleasure. The ability to react with adequate emotion to circumstances or people is reduced
0	Normal interest in the surroundings and in other people
1	
2	Reduced ability to enjoy usual interests
3	
4	Loss of interest in the surroundings. Loss of feelings for friends and acquaintances
5	
6	The experience of being emotionally paralyzed, inability to feel anger, grief or pleasure and a complete or even painful failure to feel for close relatives and friends

Montgomery-Åsberg Depression Rating Scale (continued overleaf)

Montgomery-Åsberg Depression Rating Scale (continued)

9. Pessimistic Thoughts	
	Representing thoughts of guilt, inferiority, self-reproach, sinfulness, remorse, and ruin
0	No pessimistic thoughts
1	
2	Fluctuating ideas of failure, self-reproach or self-depreciation
3	
4	Persistent self-accusations or definite but still rational ideas of guilt or sin. Increasingly pessimistic about the future
5	
6	Delusions of ruin, remorse, or irredeemable sin. Self-accusations which are absurd and unshakable
10. Suicidal Thoughts	
	Representing the feeling that life is not worth living, that a natural death would be welcome, suicidal thoughts, and preparations for suicide. Suicide attempts should not in themselves influence the rating
0	Enjoys life or takes it as it comes
1	
2	Weary of life. Only fleeting suicidal thoughts
3	
4	Probably better off dead. Suicidal thoughts are common, and suicide is considered as a possible solution, but without specific plans or intentions
5	
6	Explicit plans for suicide when there is an opportunity. Active preparations for suicide

Montgomery-Åsberg Depression Rating Scale. Reproduced with permission from Montgomery SA, Åsberg M. A new depression scale designed to be sensitive to change. *Br J Psychiatry*. 1979;134:382-389 ©Royal College of Psychiatrists.

Appendix C

The Hospital Anxiety and Depression Scale

The Hospital Anxiety and Depression Scale

A		**I feel tense or 'wound up':**
	3	Most of the time
	2	A lot of the time
	1	From time to time, occasionally
	0	Not at all
D		**I still enjoy the things I used to enjoy:**
	0	Definitely as much
	1	Not quite so much
	2	Only a little
	3	Hardly at all
A		**I get a sort of frightened feeling as if something awful is about to happen:**
	3	Very definitely and quite badly
	2	Yes, but not too badly
	1	A little, but it doesn't worry me
	0	Not at all
D		**I can laugh and see the funny side of things:**
	0	As much as I always could
	1	Not quite so much now
	2	Definitely not so much now
	3	Not at all

The Hospital Anxiety and Depression Scale (continued overleaf)

© Springer International Publishing Switzerland 2014
G. Alexopoulos et al., *Guide to Assessment Scales in Major Depressive Disorder*,
DOI 10.1007/978-3-319-04627-3

The Hospital Anxiety and Depression Scale (continued)

	A	Worrying thoughts go through my mind:
	3	A great deal of the time
	2	A lot of the time
	1	From time to time but not too often
	0	Only occasionally
D		**I feel cheerful:**
3		Not at all
2		Not often
1		Sometimes
0		Most of the time
	A	**I can sit at ease and feel relaxed:**
	0	Definitely
	1	Usually
	2	Not often
	3	Not at all
D		**I feel as if I am slowed down:**
3		Nearly all the time
2		Very often
1		Sometimes
0		Not at all
	A	**I get a sort of frightened feeling like 'butterflies' in the stomach:**
	0	Not at all
	1	Occasionally
	2	Quite often
	3	Very often
D		**I have lost interest in my appearance:**
3		Definitely
2		I don't take so much care as I should
1		I may not take quite as much care
0		I take just as much care as ever

The Hospital Anxiety and Depression Scale (continued opposite)

The Hospital Anxiety and Depression Scale (continued)

	A	I feel restless as if I have to be on the move:
	3	Very much indeed
	2	Quite a lot
	1	Not very much
	0	Not at all
D		I look forward with enjoyment to things:
0		As much as ever I did
1		Rather less than I used to
2		Definitely less than I used to
3		Hardly at all
	A	I get sudden feelings of panic:
	3	Very often indeed
	2	Quite often
	1	Not very often
	0	Not at all
D		I can enjoy a good book or radio or TV programme:
0		Often
1		Sometimes
2		Not often
3		Very seldom

Now check you have answered all questions

FOR HOSPITAL USE ONLY

D (8-10) _____

A (8-10) _____

The Hospital Anxiety and Depression Scale. *Instructions:* Doctors are aware that emotions play an important part in most illnesses. If your doctor knows about these feelings he will be able to help you more. This questionnaire is designed to help your doctor to know how you feel. Ignore the numbers printed on the left of the questionnaire. Read each item and underline the reply which comes closest to how you have been feeling in the past week. Don't take too long over your replies; your immediate reaction to each item will probably be more accurate than a long thought out response. Reproduced with permission from Zigmond AS, Snaith RP. The hospital anxiety and depression scale. *Acta Psychiatr Scand.* 1983;67:361-370 ©Wiley.

Appendix D

The Cornell Scale for Depression in Dementia

The Cornell Scale for Depression in Dementia

A. Mood-related symptoms	Informant			Patient			Rater's Opinion		
1. Anxiety Anxious expression, ruminations, worrying	0	1	2	0	1	2	0	1	2
2. Sadness Sad expression, sad voice, tearfulness	0	1	2	0	1	2	0	1	2
3. Lack of reactivity to pleasant events	0	1	2	0	1	2	0	1	2
4. Irritability Easily annoyed, short tempered	0	1	2	0	1	2	0	1	2
B. Behavioral disturbance									
5. Agitation Restlessness, handwringing, hair pulling	0	1	2	0	1	2	0	1	2
6. Retardation Slow movements, slow speech, slow reactions	0	1	2	0	1	2	0	1	2
7. Multiple physical complaints (score 0 if GI symptoms only)	0	1	2	0	1	2	0	1	2
8. Loss of interest Less involved in usual activities (score only if change occurred acutely; ie, in less than 1 month)	0	1	2	0	1	2	0	1	2
C. Physical signs									
9. Appetite loss Eating less than usual	0	1	2	0	1	2	0	1	2

The Cornell Scale for Depression in Dementia (continued overleaf)

© Springer International Publishing Switzerland 2014
G. Alexopoulos et al., *Guide to Assessment Scales in Major Depressive Disorder*,
DOI 10.1007/978-3-319-04627-3

The Cornell Scale for Depression in Dementia (continued)

	Informant			Patient			Rater's Opinion		
10. Weight loss (score 2 if greater than 5 lbs in 1 month)	0	1	2	0	1	2	0	1	2
11. Lack of energy Fatigues easily, unable to sustain activities (score only if change occurred acutely; ie, in less than 1 month)	0	1	2	0	1	2	0	1	2
D. Cyclic functions									
12. Diurnal varation of mood Symptoms worse in the morning	0	1	2	0	1	2	0	1	2
13. Difficulty falling asleep Later than usual for this individual	0	1	2	0	1	2	0	1	2
14. Multiple awakenings during sleep	0	1	2	0	1	2	0	1	2
15. Early morning awakening Earlier than usual for this individual	0	1	2	0	1	2	0	1	2
E. Ideation disturbance									
16. Suicide Feels life is not worth living, has suicidal wishes, or make suicide attempt	0	1	2	0	1	2	0	1	2
17. Self-deprecation Self-blame, poor self-esteem, feelings of failure	0	1	2	0	1	2	0	1	2
18. Pessimism Anticipation of the worst	0	1	2	0	1	2	0	1	2
19. Mood congruent delusions Delusions of poverty, illness, or loss	0	1	2	0	1	2	0	1	2
Total score:									

Reproduced with permission from Alexopoulos G et al [1] ©Elsevier.

The Cornell Scale for Depression in Dementia Guidelines

Administration and scoring

The Cornell Scale for Depression in Dementia (CSDD) was specifically developed to assess signs and symptoms of major depression in demented patients. Because some of these patients may give unreliable reports, the CSDD uses a comprehensive interviewing approach that derives information from the patient and the informant. Information is elicited through two semi-structured interviews; an interview of an informant and an interview of the patient. The interviewer should assign preliminary scores to each item of the scale on the basis of the informant's report in the "Informant" column. The next step is for the rater to interview the patient using the Cornell scale items as a guide. The interviews focus on depressive symptoms and signs occurring during the week preceding the interview. Many of the items during the patient interview can be filled after direct observation of the patient. If there are discrepancies in ratings from the informant and the patient interviews, the rater should re-interview both the informant and the patient with the goal to resolve the discrepancies. The final ratings of the CSDD items represent the rater's clinical impression rather than the responses of the informant or the patient. The CSDD takes approximately 20 minutes to administer.

Each item is rated for severity on a scale of 0–2 (0=absent, 1=mild or intermittent, 2=severe). The item scores are added. Scores above 10 indicate a probable major depression. Scores above 18 indicate a definite major depression. Scores below 6 as a rule are associated with absence of significant depressive symptoms.

Interview with the informant

Who qualifies as an Informant? Informants should know and have frequent contact with the patient. Reliable informants can include nursing staff for patients in the hospital and nursing homes or a family member for outpatients.

The informant interview should be conducted first. The interviewer should ask about any change in symptoms of depression over the previous week. The rater should complete each item on the scale. The rater can expand on the descriptions of the symptoms in order to help the informant understand each item.

For the following questions, please refer to how your relative has been feeling during the past week. Two items, item 8 ("loss of interest") and item 11 ("lack of energy"), require both: 1) a disturbance occurring during the week prior to the interview; and 2) changes in these areas have been occurring over less than one month. In these two items, the caregiver is instructed to report on the patient's behavior during the week prior to the interview and then to give the history of the onset of changes in these two areas that may have taken place at an earlier time.

A. Mood-Related Signs

1. Anxiety: *(anxious expression, ruminations, worrying)* Has your relative been feeling anxious this past week? Has s/he been worrying about things s/he may not ordinarily worry about, or ruminating over things that may not be that important? Has your relative had an anxious, tense, distressed or apprehensive expression?

2. Sadness: *(sad expression, sad voice, tearfulness)* Has your relative been feeling down, sad, or blue this past week? Has s/he been crying at all? How many days out of the past week has s/he been feeling like this? For how long each day?

3. Lack of reactivity to pleasant events: If a pleasant event were to occur today (ie, going out with spouse, friends, seeing grandchildren), would your relative be able to enjoy it fully, or might his/her mood get in the way of his/her interest in the event or activity? Does your relative's mood affect any of the following:

- his/her ability to enjoy activities that used to give him/her pleasure?
- his/her surroundings?
- his/her feelings for family and friends?

4. Irritability: *(easily annoyed, short-tempered)* Has your relative felt short-tempered or easily annoyed this past week? Has s/he been feeling irritable, impatient, or angry this week?

B. Behavioral Disturbance

5. Agitation: *(restlessness, hand-wringing, hair-pulling)* Has your relative been fidgety or restless this past week that s/he was unable to sit still for at least an hour?

Was your relative so physically agitated that you or others noticed it? Agitation may include such behaviors as playing with one's hands, hair, hand-wringing, hair-pulling, and/or lip-biting: Have you observed any such behavior in your relative during the past week?

6. Retardation: *(slow movements, slow speech, slow reactions)* Has your relative been talking or moving more slowly than is normal for him/her? This may include:

- slowness of thoughts and speech
- delayed response to your questions
- decreased motor activity and/or reactions

7. Multiple physical complaints: In the past week, has your relative had any of the following physical symptoms? (in excess of what is normal for him/her):

- indigestion?
- constipation?
- diarrhea?
- stomach cramps?
- belching?
- heart palpitations?
- headaches?
- muscles aches?
- joint pain?
- backache?
- hyperventilation (shortness of breath)?
- frequent urinations?
- sweating?

If yes to any of the above, how much have these things been bothering your relative? How bad have they become and how often have they occurred in the past week? Do not rate symptoms that are side effects from taking medications or those that are only related to GI ailments.

8. Loss of interest: *(less involved in usual activities – score only if change occurred acutely, or in less than one month)* How has your relative been spending his/her time this past week (not including work and chores)? Has your relative felt interested in his/her usual activities and hobbies? Has your relative spent any *less* time engaging in these activities?

If s/he is not as interested, or has not been that engaged in activities during the past week: Has your relative had to push him/herself to do the things s/he normally enjoys? Has your relative *stopped* doing anything s/he used to do? Can s/he look forward to anything or has s/he lost interest in many of the hobbies from which s/he used to derive pleasure?

Ratings of this item should be based on loss of interest during the past week. This item should be rated 0 if the loss of interest is long-standing (longer than 1 month) and there has been no worsening during the past month. This item should be rated 0 if the patient has not been engaged in activities because of physical illness or disability, or if the patient has persistent apathy associated with dementia.

C. Physical Signs

9. Appetite loss: *(eating less than usual)* How has your relative's appetite been this past week compared to normal? Has it decreased at all? Has your relative felt less hungry or had to remind him/herself to eat? Have others had to urge or force him/her to eat?
 – Rate 1 if there is appetite loss but still s/he is eating on his/her own.
 – Rate 2 if eats only with others' encouragement or urging.

10. Weight loss: Has your relative lost any weight in the past month that s/he has not meant to or been trying to lose? (If not sure: are your relative's clothes any looser on him/her?) If weight loss is associated with present illness (ie, not due to diet or exercise): how many pounds has s/he lost?
 – Rate 2 if weight loss is greater than 5 pounds in past month.

11. Lack of energy: *(fatigues easily, unable to sustain activities – score only if change occurred acutely, or in less than one month)* How has your relative's energy been this past week compared to normal? Has s/he been tired all the time? Has s/he asked to take naps because of fatigue? This week, has your relative had any of the following symptoms due to lack of energy only (*not due to physical problems*):
 • heaviness in limbs, back, or head?
 • felt like s/he is dragging through the day?
Has your relative been fatigued more easily this week?
 – Ratings of this item should be based on lack of energy during the week prior to the interview. This item should be rated 0 if the lack of energy is long-standing (longer than 1 month) and there has been no worsening during the past month.

D. Cyclic Functions

12. Diurnal variation of mood: *(symptoms worse in the morning)* Regarding your relative's mood (his/her feelings and symptoms of depression), is there any part of the day in which s/

he usually feels better or worse? (or does it not make any difference, or vary according to the day or situation?)
 - If yes to a difference in mood during the day: Is your relative's depression worse in the morning or the evening?
 - If worse in the morning: Is this a mild or a very noticeable difference?

S/he must consistently feel worse in the mornings (as compared to evenings) for this item to be rated.

Diurnal variation of mood is only rated for symptoms that are worse in the morning. Variation of mood in the evening can be related to sun downing in patients with dementia and should not be rated.

13. Difficulty falling asleep: *(later than usual for this individual)* Has your relative had any trouble falling asleep this past week? Does it take him/her longer than usual to fall asleep once s/he gets into bed (ie, more than 30 min)?
 - Rate 1 if patient only had trouble falling asleep a few nights in the past week.
 - Rate 2 if s/he has had difficulty falling asleep every night this past week.

14. Multiple awakenings during sleep: Has your relative been waking up in the middle of the night this past week? If yes: does s/he get out of bed? Is this just to go to the bathroom and then s/he goes back to sleep?
 - Do not rate if waking is only to go to the bathroom and then is able to fall right back asleep.
 - Rate 1 if sleep has only been restless and disturbed occasionally in the past week, and has not gotten out of bed (besides going to the bathroom).
 - Rate 2 if s/he gets out of bed in the middle of the night (for reasons other than voiding), and/or has been waking up every night in the past week.

15. Early morning awakenings: *(earlier than usual for this individual)* Has your relative been waking up any earlier this week than s/he normally does (without an alarm clock or someone waking him/her up)? If yes: how much earlier is s/he waking up than is normal for him/her? Does your relative get out of bed when s/he wakes up early, or does s/he stay in bed and/or go back to sleep?
 - Rate 1 if s/he wakes up on his/her own but then goes back to sleep.
 - Rate 2 if s/he wakes earlier than usual and then gets out of bed for the day (ie, s/he cannot fall back asleep).

E. Ideational Disturbance

16. Suicide: *(feels life is not worth living, has suicidal wishes, or makes suicide attempt)* During the past week, has your relative had any thoughts that life is not worth living or that s/he would be better off dead? Has s/he had any thoughts of hurting or even killing him/herself?
 - Rate 1 for passive suicidal ideation (ie, feels life isn't worth living).
 - Rate 2 for active suicidal wishes, and/or any recent suicide attempts, gestures, or plans.

History of suicide attempt in a subject with no passive or active suicidal ideation does not in itself justify a score.

17. Self-depreciation: *(self-blame, poor self-esteem, feelings of failure)* How has your relative been feeling about him/herself this past week? Has s/he been feeling especially critical of him/herself, feeling that s/he has done things wrong or let others down? Has s/he been feeling guilty about anything s/he has or has not done? Has s/he been comparing him/herself to others, or feeling worthless, or like a failure? Has s/he described him/herself as "no good" or "inferior"?

– Rate 1 for loss of self-esteem or self-reproach.
– Rate 2 for feelings of failure, or statements that s/he is "worthless," "inferior," or "no good."

18. Pessimism: *(anticipation of the worst)* Has your relative felt pessimistic or discouraged about his/her future this past week? Can your relative see his/her situation improving? Can your relative be reassured by others that things will be okay or that his/her situation will improve?

– Rate 1 if s/he feels pessimistic, but can be reassured by self or others.
– Rate 2 if feels hopeless and cannot be reassured that his/her future will be okay.

19. Mood congruent delusions: *(delusions of poverty, illness, or loss)* Has your relative been having ideas that others may find strange? Does your relative think his/her present illness is a punishment, or that s/he has brought it on him/herself in some irrational way? Does your relative think s/he has less money or material possessions than s/he really does?

Interview with the patient

Ratings of most Patient Interview items should be principally based on direct observation. Questions to the patient may offer supplemental information or be the main reference to how you have been feeling during the past week.

A. Mood Related Signs:

1. Anxiety: *(anxious expression, ruminations, worrying)* Does the subject have an anxious, tense, distressed or apprehensive expression?

Ask the patient: Have you been feeling anxious this past week? Have you been worrying about things you may not ordinarily worry about, or ruminating over things that may not be that important?

2. Sadness: *(sad expression, sad voice, tearfulness)* Does the patient have a sad expression or sad voice? Is the patient tearful?

Ask the patient: Have you been feeling down, sad, or blue this past week? Have you been crying at all? How many days out of the past week have you been feeling like this? For how long each day?

3. Lack of reactivity to pleasant events: Is the patient able to respond to friendly or supportive remarks or to humor?

Ask the patient: If a pleasant event were to occur today (ie, going out with your spouse, friends, seeing your grandchildren), would you be able to enjoy it fully, or might your mood get in the way of your interest in the event or activity? Does your mood affect any of the following:

- your ability to enjoy activities that used to give you pleasure?
- your surroundings?
- your feelings for your family and friends?

4. Irritability: *(easily annoyed, short tempered)* Observe whether the patient is easily annoyed and short-tempered during the interview.

Ask the patient: Have you felt short-tempered or easily annoyed this past week? Have you been feeling irritable, impatient, or angry this week?

B. Behavioral Disturbance

5. Agitation *(restlessness, hand-wringing, hair-pulling):* Observe the patient for behaviors such as playing with his/her hands, hair, hand-wringing, hair-pulling, and/or lip-biting.

Ask the patient: Have you been fidgety or restless this past week? Have you been unable to sit still for at least an hour? Were you so physically agitated to the point that others noticed it?

6. Retardation: *(slow movements, slow speech, slow reactions)* This item should be scored *exclusively on the basis of the rater's observations.* Retardation is characterized by:

- slow speech
- delayed response to questions
- decreased motor activity and/or reactions

7. Multiple physical complaints: In the past week, have you had any of the following physical symptoms in excess to what is normal for you:

- indigestion?
- constipation?
- diarrhea?
- stomach cramps?
- belching?
- heart palpitations?
- headaches?
- muscle aches?
- joint pain?
- backache?
- hyperventilation (shortness of breath)?
- frequent urination?
- sweating?

If yes to any of the above: How much have these things been bothering you? How bad have they gotten and how often have they occurred in the past week?

- – Do not rate symptoms that are side effects from taking medications or those that are only related to gastrointestinal ailments.

8. Loss of interest: *(less involved in usual activities – score only if change occurred acutely, or in less than one month)* How have you been spending your time this past week (not including work and chores)? Have you felt interested in what you usually like to do? Have you spent any *less* time engaging in these activities?

If not as interested, or has not been engaged in activities during the past week: Have you had to push yourself to do the things you normally enjoy? Have you *stopped* doing anything you used to do? Can you look forward to anything or have you lost interest in many of the hobbies from which you used to derive pleasure?

Ratings of this item should be based on loss of interest during the past week. This item should be rated 0 if the loss of interest is long-standing (longer than 1 month) and there has been no worsening during the past month. This item should be rated 0, if the patient has not been engaged in activities because of physical illness or disability or if the patient has persistent apathy as part of his/her dementia.

C. Physical Signs

9. Appetite Loss: *(eating less than usual)* How has your appetite been this past week compared to normal? Has it decreased at all? Have you felt less hungry or had to remind yourself to eat? Have others had to urge or force you to eat?
  − Rate 1 if appetite loss but still eating on his/her own.
  − Rate 2 if eats only with others' encouragement or urging.

10. Weight Loss: Have you lost any weight in the past month that you have not been trying to lose? (If not sure: are your clothes any looser on you?) If weight loss is associated with present illness (ie, not due to diet or exercise): how many pounds have you lost?
  − Rate 2 if weight loss is greater than 5 lbs. in past month.

11. Lack of energy: *(fatigues easily, unable to sustain activities – score only if change occurred acutely, or in less than one month)* Does the patient appear fatigued or drained of energy?

Ask the patient: How has your energy been this past week compared to normal? Have you been tired all the time? Have you needed to take naps because of fatigue? Have you any of the following symptoms due to lack of energy only (*not* due to physical problems):
  • heaviness in limbs, back, or head?
  • felt like you are dragging through the day?
  − Ratings of this item should be based on lack of energy during the week prior to the interview. This item should be rated 0 if the lack of energy is longstanding (longer than 1 month) and there has been no worsening during the past month.

D. Cyclic Functions

12. Diurnal variation of mood: *(symptoms worse in the morning)* Regarding your mood (feelings and symptoms of depression), is there any part of the day in which you usually feel better or worse? (Or does it not make any difference, or vary according to the day or situation?)

- If yes to a difference in mood during the day: Is your depression worse in the morning or the evening?
- If worse in the morning: is this a mild or a very noticeable difference?

The subject must feel consistently worse in the mornings (as compared to evenings) for this item to be rated.

Diurnal variation of mood is only rated for symptoms that are worse in the morning. Variation of mood in the evening can be related to sun downing in patients with dementia and should not be rated.

13. Difficulty falling asleep: *(later than usual for this individual)* Have you had any trouble falling asleep this past week? Does it take you longer than usual to fall asleep once you get into bed (ie, more than 30 min)?
- Rate 1 if only the subject had trouble falling asleep a few nights in the past week.
- Rate 2 if s/he has had difficulty falling asleep every night this past week.

14. Multiple awakenings during sleep: Have you been waking up in the middle of the night this past week more than usual? If yes: do you get out of bed? Is this just to go to the bathroom and then you go back to sleep?
- Do not rate if waking is only to go to the bathroom and then is able to fall right back asleep.
- Rate 1 if sleep has only been restless and disturbed occasionally in the past week, and has not gotten out of bed (besides going to the bathroom).
- Rate 2 if s/he gets out of bed in the middle of the night (for reasons other than voiding), and/or has been waking up every night in the past week.

15. Early morning awakenings: *(earlier than usual for this individual)* Have you been waking up any earlier this week than you normally do (without an alarm clock or someone waking you up)? If yes: how much earlier are you waking up than is normal for you? Do you get out of bed when you wake up early, or do you stay in bed and/or go back to sleep?
- Rate 1 if s/he wakes up on his/her own but then goes back to sleep.
- Rate 2 if s/he wakes earlier than usual and then gets out of bed for the day (ie, s/he cannot fall back asleep).

E. Ideational Disturbance

16. Suicide: *(feels life is not worth living, has suicidal wishes, or makes suicide attempt)* During the past week, have you had any thoughts that life is not worth living or that you would be better off dead? Have you had any thoughts of hurting or even killing yourself?
- Rate 1 for passive suicidal ideation (ie, feels life isn't worth living).
- Rate 2 for active suicidal wishes, and/or any recent suicide attempts, gestures, or plans. History of suicide attempt in a subject with no passive or active suicidal ideation does not in itself justify a score.

17. Self-depreciation: *(self-blame, poor self esteem, feelings of failure)* How have you been feeling about yourself this past week? Have you been feeling especially critical of yourself, feeling that you have done things wrong or let others down? Have you been feeling guilty about anything you have or have not done? Have you been comparing yourself to others, or feeling worthless, or like a failure? Have you felt "no good" or "inferior"?

- Rate 1 for loss of self-esteem or self-reproach.
- Rate 2 for feelings of failure, or statements that s/he is "worthless," "inferior," or "no good."

18. Pessimism: *(anticipation of the worst)* Have you felt pessimistic or discouraged about your future this past week? How do you think things will work out for yourself? Can you see your situation improving? Can you be reassured by others that things will be okay or that your situation will improve?

- Rate 1 if s/he feels pessimistic, but can be reassured by self or others.
- Rate 2 if feels hopeless and cannot be reassured that his/her future will be okay.

19. Mood congruent delusions: *(delusions of poverty, illness, or loss)* Have you been seeing or hearing things that others do not see or hear? Has your imagination been playing tricks on you in any way, or have you been having ideas that others may not understand? Do you think that your present illness is a punishment, or that you have brought it on yourself in some way? Do you think you have a lot less money or material possessions than others say that you have?

Reproduced with permission from Alexopoulos GA, Abrams RC, Young RC, Shamoian CA. Cornell scale for depression in dementia. *Biol Psych*. 1988;23:271-284. ©Elsevier.